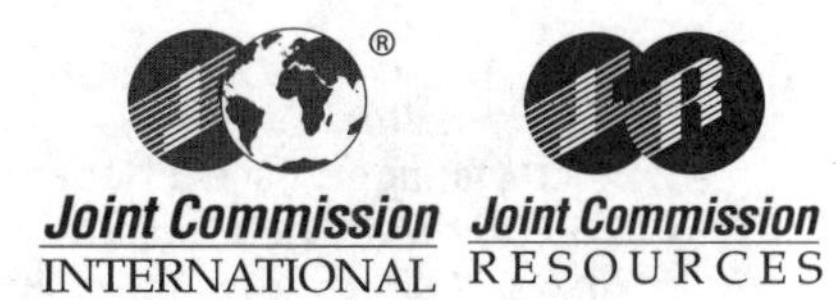

BEST PRACTICES IN INFECTION CONTROL

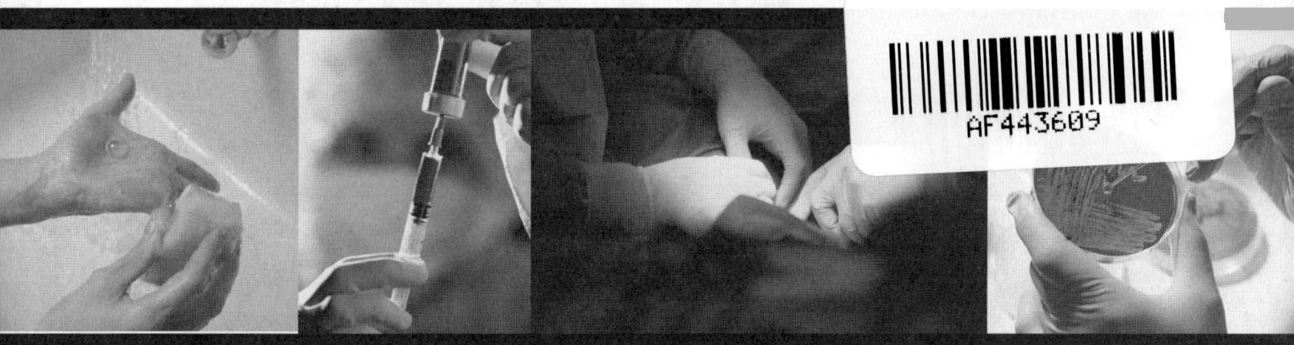

AN INTERNATIONAL HANDBOOK

EDITED BY

BARBARA M. SOULE, R.N., M.P.A., CIC

PROF. ZIAD A. MEMISH, M.D., FRCPC, FACP, CIC, FIDSA

Executive Editor: Paul Reis
Project Manager: Rachel Hegarty
Production Manager: Johanna Harris
Manager, Publications: Diane Bell
Associate Director: Cecily Pew
Executive Director: Catherine Chopp Hinckley
Vice President, Learning: Charles Macfarlane, FACHE
Joint Commission/JCI Reviewers: Diane Bell, Cecily Pew, Maureen Potter, Anne Rooney, Paul vanOstenberg, Richard Croteau
Other Reviewers: Patricia Lynch, R.N., M.B.A.; Nizam Damani, M.D., MBBS, MSc, FRCPI, FRCPath
Content Editors:

Barbara M. Soule, R.N., M.P.A., CIC
Practice Leader, Infection Prevention and Control Services
Joint Commission Resources
Joint Commission International

Prof. Ziad A. Memish, M.D., FRCPC, FACP, CIC, FIDSA
Chief, Adult Infectious Diseases, Department of Medicine
Executive Director, Infection Prevention and Control Program
King Abdulaziz Medical City
King Fahad National Guard Hospital
National Guard Health Affairs
Riyadh, Saudi Arabia
Adjunct Professor, Department of Medicine, Division of Infectious Diseases
Ottawa University
Ottawa, Ontario, Canada

Joint Commission International
The mission of Joint Commission International is to improve the quality of care in the international community through the provision of education and consultation services.

Joint Commission Resources educational programs and publications support, but are separate from, the accreditation activities of Joint Commission International. Attendees at Joint Commission Resources educational programs and purchasers of Joint Commission Resources publications receive no special consideration or treatment in, or confidential information about, the accreditation process.

Printed in the U.S.A. 5 4 3 2 1

Requests for permission to make copies of any part of this work should be mailed to

Permissions Editor
Department of Publications
Joint Commission Resources
One Renaissance Boulevard
Oakbrook Terrace, Illinois 60181
permissions@jcrinc.com

ISBN 13: 978-0-86688-965-0 (softcover)   978-1-59940-030-3 (hardcover)
ISBN 10:   0-86688-965-5 (softcover)   1-59940-030-8 (hardcover)
Library of Congress Control Number: 2006935456

For more information about Joint Commission Resources, please visit http://www.jcrinc.com.

Contents

Foreword

Like all human beings, I am always a potential patient. So I am interested in the safety of the setting in which health care is delivered, and particularly in the risk of acquiring infections in those settings. The more I learn about this latter risk, the more anxious I get. Over the past century, effective vaccines, new technological capabilities, and powerful antibiotics, have had significant impacts on preventing, controlling, and curing certain infections. But the fact is that the infectious risks we face today are potentially as lethal as anything we have ever faced before.

Here are some of the hard realities: The World Health Organization estimates that at least one in four patients treated in intensive care units around the world will acquire an infection during their hospital stay. In developing countries, those numbers may be two of four patients. In the United States alone, there are two million hospital-acquired infections per year; some Centers for Disease Control and Prevention staff say that number may be closer to four million. These infections lead to at least ninety thousand deaths per year. The actual number may be substantially more than that, but it is probably not less. At least a third of these deaths are preventable. On a proportionate basis, there is no evidence that this situation is any better anywhere else in the world.

On top of this and more broadly, we face the risks of emerging infections, like HIV/AIDS once was and like SARS was, in more recent memory. We have old infections, but only partially effective vaccines or insufficient amounts of effective vaccines. And then there are the risks of bioterrorism, where effective detection and protection are almost imponderables. Herein also lies the risk of contamination of facilities and staff and the resulting disabling of major segments of the care delivery system. Finally, we have the potential lethality of diseases that do not go away to eventually overwhelm the system, such as HIV/AIDS, tuberculosis, and malaria.

There is no safe place. These problems know no national boundaries. While the infection prevention and control issues and challenges vary across the spectrum of developed transitional and underdeveloped countries, certain common themes are identifiable, such as inadequate attention, indeed inadequate commitment, to simple hand washing. Effective hand washing remains the single most important preventive measure we know of. It is bad enough that patients, or simply just the public, are not constantly reminded about the why and the how of hand washing, but it is far worse that health care professionals—"the teachers"—are so cavalier about washing their own hands. These latter individuals have become some of the worst vectors known to man for transmitting serious infectious diseases. Further, some of these practitioners are the same professionals whose misuse of antibiotics leads to the emergence of drug-resistant microorganisms, which they, among others, then help to transmit to patients as a consequence of inadequate hand hygiene—not an attractive picture.

And these are not the only challenges. Infections are acquired by many routes. Cleanliness issues exist and continue to arise regarding medications, vaccines, intravenous fluids, blood, and other therapeutic products. These challenges exist even in sophisticated, developed countries. There are also challenges regarding the cleanliness of equipment. In underdeveloped countries, we are often talking about clean needles and syringes. But in developed countries, we are talking about inadequate cleaning of endoscopes and ventilators and even failed instrument sterilization, which, for example, raises the specter of mad cow disease.

The performance of clean surgical procedures is also an issue. Here, aseptic technique is certainly important, but so too is the appropriate and timely use of prophylactic antibiotics. Such antibiotic use acknowledges some of the vulnerabilities inherent in current techniques and the resulting risks to patients. The commonplace insertion of central lines and the resulting risk of bloodstream infections is a similar problem.

Finally, we face the challenges of maintaining a clean environment and assuring continuing access to clean water. Effective health-waste disposal is a problem in underdeveloped countries, and, I would hasten to add, in developed countries as well. That would include our home city of Chicago among other places. The issue of clean water is even more compelling, because washing your hands does not do much good if you are using dirty water. Dirty water is a problem everywhere, including the United States at times.

These challenges exist everywhere. Only the form of the problem varies from country to country and from setting to setting. What needs to be done?

First of all, we need to be paying a lot more attention to systems design—or very simply put, "how we do things here." Infections are not inevitable. They do not just happen. They can be prevented. But people who provide care need to know a lot more about how to design "how we do things here" to keep infections from reaching patients, to keep errors of all kinds from reaching patients. And that means developing a capability for systems analysis and systems redesign across health care settings to achieve those fundamental ends.

Coupled with that has to be an intervention mindset. To this time, we have paid much more attention to surveillance and gathering data about trends and far too little attention to intervening—to analyzing the case of the single patient who should have walked out of the hospital safely but instead acquired an infection and died, to learning what systems changes might have prevented that infection, and to acting to make those changes. That one case is a real human being and he or she did not need to die. We owe that intervention mindset to these patients.

We also need to create solutions that are workable and easy to implement. Solutions that distract practitioners from their usual work and whose benefits are not readily apparent will not achieve adoption on a scale necessary to reduce infection risks.

Thought also needs to be given to creating forcing functions. *Forcing function* is a technical term, but to illustrate by fantasy, it would be as if some invisible shield prevented a practitioner from touching a patient unless the practitioner had washed his or her hands. Or maybe the simplest thing is to make sure that patients ask practitioners every time, "Did you wash your hands?"

There are, additionally, issues of organization leadership. Whether in charge of big organizations or small, leaders everywhere need to place a high priority on infection prevention and control. It is they, for instance, who control the deployment of scarce resources that may be desperately needed to reduce infection risk. Leaders also need to be willing to make unpopular decisions—such as closing a contaminated nursery—because that is what leadership is all about.

We also need competent practitioners. No organization is any better at reducing infection risk than the quality of its infection prevention and control practitioner. That is a fundamental truth. All countries need to be sure that they are investing in adequate numbers of properly trained practitioners as a top priority.

We further need a measurement capability to know how we are doing. This can be challenging because there are two key variables at play—the actual number of hospital-acquired infections and the skill of the infection prevention and control practitioner in identifying cases. Thus, organizations that are good case finders have higher infection rates, and organizations that are poor case finders are more likely to have low rates. This makes it difficult to judge the quality of the organization's quality control efforts per se, a problem now compounded by growing pressure to publicly report organization infection rates.

Finally, the most important thing we need to do is to create cultures of safety in health care organizations. It is one thing to create expectations, either as an accreditor such as we are or ministry of health in another country, but it is quite another to make them happen. The solutions I have described will be put in place when organizations begin to "own" them. These solutions need to matter to these organizations and their leaders.

And we all need to come to a clear understanding that there is a problem, that it is a serious problem, and that it is our problem. Then it will become a solvable problem, one commitment and one step at a time.

Dennis S. O'Leary, M.D.
President, Joint Commission on
Accreditation of Healthcare Organizations

Introduction

In today's health care environment, organizations are challenged with a multitude of infection prevention and control (IPC) issues. Health care–associated infections, resource and infrastructure limitations, outbreaks, emerging and reemerging diseases, and threat of pandemics or bioterrorism make IPC a priority in health care settings across the spectrum of care. This book focuses on the growing crisis in IPC and outlines Joint Commission International's (JCI's) requirements for meeting accreditation standards. It offers health care leaders, IPC specialists, and other health care providers ideas for improvement and shares valuable lessons learned from a variety of organizations.

After reading this book, health care organizations will be able to do the following:

- Discuss some of the current and future IPC challenges in health care organizations and communities throughout the world
- Describe the JCI requirements in the area of IPC, including the new Prevention and Control of Infections (PCI) standards and the International Patient Safety Goal relating to IPC
- Proactively evaluate their own compliance with JCI requirements and identify areas for improvement
- Apply practical tips and evidence-based information to their own IPC program, planning, and efforts
- Incorporate in their own IPC, patient safety, and quality improvement activities lessons learned from real-world examples and case studies

The Content

Chapter 1—Infection Prevention and Control:
A Global Perspective on a Health Care Crisis
This chapter discusses the field of IPC from a global perspective, including present challenges and those on the horizon. It discusses health care–associated infections, emerging and reemerging infectious diseases in the communities and the health care settings and infectious diseases associated with bioterrorism. The chapter also takes a brief look at what JCI and other international organizations are doing to help health care organizations address IPC issues.

*Chapter 2—Joint Commission International's Infection
Prevention and Control Standards and Requirements: A Detailed Study*
This chapter takes an in-depth look at the new and revised PCI standards for ambulatory care, hospitals, clinical laboratories, and medical transport organizations. It also examines the International Patient Safety Goals, specifically the goal dealing with hand hygiene, and the reporting of infection-related adverse events.

Chapter 3—Surveying Infection Prevention and Control
This chapter walks organizations through the accreditation process as it relates to IPC, including how surveyors survey the standards and the International Patient Safety Goal.

*Chapter 4—Developing an Effective Infection Prevention
and Control Program: Challenges, Tips, and Tools for Success*
The effective IPC program can be challenging to create. This chapter discusses some of the challenges of assessing risk and developing goals and objectives and workable infection prevention plans. It also offers suggestions and tips to help organizations with these IPC efforts. Brief case studies from organizations around the country and some tools offer real-world examples and provide lessons learned.

*Chapter 5—Maintaining an Effective Infection Prevention
and Control Program: More Challenges, Tips, and Tools*
After an organization creates an IPC program, it should put into place certain interventions to maintain its effectiveness, including programs for hand hygiene, device safety, sterilization and disinfection, and emergency preparedness. This chapter also discusses some of the challenges in creating and implementing IPC interventions and offers some tips for success. The Pandemic Preparedness Project, an effort of the Royal Institution World Science Assembly, is explored in depth.

*Chapter 6—Lessons Learned:
The 2003 Hong Kong and Toronto SARS Outbreaks*
In 2003 Hong Kong and Canada experienced firsthand some of the challenges of dealing with an outbreak of a major new infectious disease. This chapter discusses what happened and offers some lessons learned that organizations can use in developing their own IPC emergency response plans.

At the end of each chapter, wide-ranging written and online resources for additional research are provided by the International Federation of Infection Control (IFIC), as compiled for that organization's forthcoming publication, *Information Resources in Infection Control,* Fourth Edition

(Editor: Nizam Damani M.D., MBBS, MSc, FRCPI, FRCPath). The full document will be available online at IFIC's Web site: http://www.theific.org/publications.asp.

Three appendixes augment the primary text—"JCI Prevention and Control of Infections Standards and Compliance Checklist" (Appendix 1); "How-to Guide: Improving Hand Hygiene, from the Institute for Healthcare Improvement" (Appendix 2); and "Infection Prevention and Control Web Resources, from the International Federation of Infection Control" (Appendix 3), which, like chapter-ending resources, is also courtesy of IFIC's *Information Resources in Infection Control,* Fourth Edition. A detailed index completes the text.

Audience

This book is intended to provide benefit for IPC and quality improvement professionals, organization leaders, clinical leaders, nursing leaders, and other staff involved in IPC in every area of health care, including ambulatory care organizations, hospitals, clinical laboratories, and medical transport organizations.

Terminology

Different health care settings use different language to refer to the individuals who receive care in their organization. This book uses the following terms:

- **Care**—also refers to treatment and services
- **Care providers**—refers to those who furnish care, treatment, and services
- **Culture of safety**—refers to an expectation or an atmosphere in which errors never or seldom occur because staff are trained to avoid practices and circumstances that produce errors
- **Endemic infections**—normal or expected incidence of infections in a population
- **Epidemic**—greater than expected number of infections in a given population during a defined period
- **Pandemic**—an epidemic (an outbreak of an infectious disease) that spreads worldwide, or at least across a large region
- **Health care settings**—refers to any location where care is provided (for example, local clinics, hospitals, long term care, temporary health delivery areas—for example, during migrations)
- **Leadership**—refers to those who set expectations, develop plans, and implement procedures; and those who manage and supervise other health care professionals, from owners to senior nurses
- **Organization**—refers to all types of organizations accredited by JCI (ambulatory care, clinical laboratory, hospital, medical transport, and those in the care continuum)

- **Outcome surveillance**—refers to examining the results of infection prevention and control processes or procedures after they are implemented and performed
- **Patient**—the individual who receives health care, treatment, and services
- **Process surveillance**—examining infection control processes or procedures before and as they are implemented
- **Safety**—the degree to which the risk of intervention and risk in the care environment are reduced for a patient and other persons, including health care providers
- **Security**—protection from loss, destruction, tampering, or unauthorized access or use

Acknowledgments

Publications of this nature are the result of the important contributions of many individuals. As a result, Joint Commission International is grateful to all of those who contributed to the success of this publication, most particularly to Dr. Dennis S. O'Leary, president of the Joint Commission on Accreditation of Healthcare Organizations, for contributing the foreword, and to the publication's content editors, Barbara M. Soule and Ziad A. Memish, for their dedication. Content reviewers Diane Bell, Richard Croteau, Nizam Damani, Candace Friedman, Patricia Lynch, Cecily Pew, Maureen Potter, Anne Rooney, and Paul vanOstenberg also contributed greatly to the finished product.

CHAPTER ONE

Infection Prevention and Control

A Global Perspective on a Health Care Crisis

Infections and infectious diseases have been around for thousands of years. They create mild to severe illness and sometimes death. Health professionals have struggled to reduce or eliminate these infections and have sometimes been successful. Yet they persist, and new infections emerge on a continual basis.

In recent years, several issues have focused public and media attention on infection prevention and control (IPC). Infections in hospitals, ambulatory care, long term care, and other health care settings have become part of the conversation of everyday life. These infections affect millions of people throughout the world and are an increasing global concern. Infectious diseases, such as severe acute respiratory syndrome (SARS), multidrug-resistant forms of tuberculosis, avian influenza, West Nile virus, dengue hemorrhagic fever, methicillin-resistant *Staphylococcus aureus* (MRSA), and vancomycin-resistant enterococci, hepatitis, and others have led international headlines and turned the public's attention to these diseases, making patients and families more aware of the possibility and danger of infection. Widespread epidemics or pandemics, emergence of highly resistant microorganisms, and infectious results of bioterrorism represent other potential threats to health care settings throughout the world.

Health Care–Associated Infections

One of the primary responsibilities of care providers and health care organizations is to do no harm to the patient. Yet, health care delivery has inherent risks. Diagnosing and treating patients often requires invasive procedures that increase infection risk. Many patients are immunocompromised, and microorganisms are becoming increasingly resistant to the available drugs. Health care organizations can be reservoirs for infections, and health care–associated illness remains an enormous factor in health care despite advanced technology, cleanliness standards, and well-intentioned staff. The safety of both patients and staff is at risk because of these infections, yet the ever-growing number of ill persons receiving treatment from health care organizations, coupled with staffing shortages or poorly trained staff, lack of supplies, and the need to reduce costs in all settings has led to increased pressure on organizations to do more with less. Over time, the lengths of stay for many hospital procedures have shortened, and care that was once limited to the acute care setting is now provided in the home, subacute and rehabilitation facilities, ambulatory clinics, and other care areas. This shift in settings has increased the risk of infection at all points along the care continuum. The serious nature of infections and the damage they can cause is undeniable. The safety risks for patients and staff are real. Health care organizations in all settings must make infection prevention and control a priority. The following sections further discuss the components of the IPC crisis and identify some challenges on the horizon.

Recent data assembled by the World Health Organization (WHO) indicate that at any time, more than 1.4 million people worldwide have infections acquired in hospitals.[1] As many as 10% of patients admitted to modern hospitals and 15% to 40% of those admitted to critical care in developed countries will acquire one or more infections.[2] One in 136 U.S. patients—which works out to 2 million cases, 80,000 deaths, and estimated additional costs of roughly US$5 billion—becomes severely ill as a result of acquiring an infection in hospital.[3] Health care–associated infections (HAIs) in England cost as much as £1 billion and more than 5,000 lives annually,[4] and in Mexico, a one-day prevalence survey in 254 adult intensive care units (ICUs) throughout the nation showed that 23% of patients in these ICUs developed HAIs.[5] More than half of all infants in developing countries' neonatal units acquire an HAI, with fatality rates ranging from 4% to an astounding 56%.[6] In 2003, during the pandemic of SARS, between 20% and 60% of health care workers caring for these patients were infected.[7,8]

Although it is true that some patients who acquire infections in a health care organization are frail, elderly, or immunocompromised, there are also healthy people who enter health care organizations for elective procedures, fully expecting to return home in good health, and instead acquire infections that sometimes result in death.[9] Unfortunately, infections pose a significant threat to patient safety, and organizations must work to prevent them when possible and mitigate their effects when prevention cannot be accomplished.

Traditionally, the spotlight for concerns about HAIs has focused predominantly on hospitals, but as care that used to be provided in hospitals becomes available in outpatient care facilities, health care organizations of all types must address a variety of different infections, including, but not limited to, the following:

- Catheter-associated urinary tract infections
- Ventilator-associated pneumonia
- Device-associated bloodstream infections
- Surgical-site infections
- Skin and soft tissue infections

The many reasons that infections occur in a health care setting include the following:

- Lack of infrastructure to support the IPC program (for example, ineffective or absent leadership support, insufficient staffing levels [*see* Sidebar 1-1] or staff training about infection and control, lack of supplies)
- Inadequate hand hygiene, aseptic or sterile technique
- The development of multidrug-resistant organisms due to the inappropriate use of antimicrobial agents
- Increasing number of immunocompromised patients
- Inappropriate or inadequate procedures and techniques of care
- Ineffective cleaning and disinfection of the patient care environment or medical equipment
- Public health issues such as contaminated water supply and inadequate management of medical waste

The keys to addressing HAIs are early detection and prevention. Organizations that implement the following practices and programs have the best chance of halting infections and reducing their transmission:

- Evidence-based hand hygiene
- Antibiotic education and monitoring
- Sufficient staffing
- Surveillance for patterns of infections and identifying areas that need specific interventions
- Infection risk reduction
- Well-educated staff

Tips on how to develop such programs appear in Chapters 4 and 5.

Emerging and Reemerging Diseases, Epidemics, and Bioterrorism

When designing programs to reduce risk of infections in health care settings, organizations must be aware of infectious diseases from the community. There is constant evolution of microorganisms, with subsequent emergence of new infections. Many serious and devastating infections ebb and flow as they reemerge in a community or a country, sometimes in more virulent forms or as epidemics. Many persons infected in the community must be hospitalized, seen in clinics, or cared for in the home by family who may then become infected. Therefore, IPC professionals in health care

SIDEBAR 1-1

The Nursing Shortage Hinders Infection Prevention and Control

Nurses have always played a crucial role in preventing the spread of infection. In today's era many health care settings lack adequate numbers of nurses, are eliminating nursing positions for cost savings or during restructuring, or do not fully train nurses in infection prevention practices.[1] At the same time more invasive devices are being used for diagnosis and treatment, patients are older or increasingly immunocompromised, new infections are emerging, and antibiotic-resistant strains are developing. The role of the nurse as the first line of defense against infection has never been more important.[2,3]

Unfortunately, the shortage of nursing professionals has contributed to the infection and prevention control (IPC) crisis throughout the world. When health care organizations operate with inadequate staff, there are increased time pressures and distractions for nurses. Critical infection prevention practices such as hand hygiene and aseptic technique are not performed consistently as staff members make choices on how to best spend the little time they have. Multiple studies have shown that inadequate nurse staffing, training, and time have contributed to health care–associated infections, such as catheter-associated primary bloodstream infection,[4] gastrointestinal illness,[5] urinary tract infections,[6] hepatitis C virus,[7] and the spread of multidrug-resistant organisms in intensive care, general wards, and burn units.[8,9] One study in a postanesthesia care unit showed that the higher a health care professional's workload, the higher the number of times hand washing was necessary, yet the lower the compliance.[10]

In many countries nurse training is minimal and staff knowledge about IPC practices is limited. This interferes with the ability to provide the safest and highest quality of care for patients. To offset the negative impact of the nursing shortage, and to enhance effective infection prevention practices, health care organizations should review their staffing policies and staff training programs and make the changes necessary to allow staff ample time to learn about and engage in appropriate IPC practices.

References

1. Hugonnet S., et. al.: Nursing resources: A major determinant of nosocomial infection? *Curr Opin Infect Dis* 17:329–333, Aug. 2004.
2. Beyea S.: Keeping patients safe from infection. *AORN J*, Jul. 2003.
3. Stone P.W., et al.: Nurses' working conditions: Implications for infectious disease. *BMJ* 321:302, Nov. 2000.
4. Fridkin S.K., et al.: The role of understaffing in central venous catheter-associated bloodstream infections. *Infect Control Hosp Epidemiol* 17:147–149, Mar. 1996.
5. Stegenga J., Bell E., Matlow A.: The role of nurse understaffing in nosocomial viral gastrointestinal infections on a general pediatrics ward. *Infect Control Hosp Epidemiol* 23:133–136, Mar. 2002.
6. Needleman J., et al.: Nurse-staffing levels and the quality of care in hospitals. *N Engl J Med* 346;22:1715–1722, May 30, 2002.
7. Saxena A.K., Panhotra, B.R.: The impact of nurse understaffing on the transmission of hepatitis C virus in a hospital-based hemodialysis unit. *Med Princ Pract* 13:129–135, May–Jun. 2004.
8. Vicca A.F.: Nursing staff workload as a determinant of methicillin-resistant *Staphylococcus aureus* spread in an adult intensive therapy unit. *J Hosp Infect*, 45:78–80, May 2000.
9. Arnow P., et. al.: Control of methicillin-resistant *Staphylococcus aureus* in a burn unit: Role of nurse staffing. *J Trauma* 22:954–959, Nov. 1982.
10. Pittet, D., et al.: Hand cleansing during post-anesthesia care. *Anesthesiology* 99:530–535, Sep. 2003.

organizations must design their IPC programs to include persons from the community who bring infections into the health care organization. Below is a discussion of selected emerging diseases that occur in the global community. Additional readings on this topic can be found at the end of this chapter.

Emerging Infectious Diseases

In 1978 the United Nations predicted that by 2000, infectious diseases would not pose a major threat to human beings even in the poorest of nations. Unfortunately, in 1998 approximately 15 million people died of infectious diseases worldwide.[10] Not only are infectious diseases not going away, but new ones are emerging. Since 1973 more than 30 new diseases have emerged that are associated with viruses or bacteria.[11]

The 2003 outbreak of a then new respiratory infection, SARS, in Asia and Canada, the introduction of West Nile virus (WNV) infections in North America, the imminently threatening avian influenza, and continuing threats from meningococcal and diarrheal diseases, dengue hemorrhagic fever, and many other serious infections point to a worldwide environment in which infectious disease continues to thrive and new strains are developing. These diseases highlight the importance of vigilance, preparedness, early identification, and open communication, to limit their effects and preserve patient safety in community and health care–delivery settings.

West Nile Virus

West Nile virus has been found in Africa, Europe, the Middle East, west and central Asia, Oceania, and North America. Outbreaks of WNV encephalitis in humans have occurred in Algeria in 1994, Romania in 1996–1997, the Czech Republic in 1997, the Democratic Republic of the Congo in 1998, Russia in 1999, Israel in 2000, and the United States in 1999 through 2003.[12] In addition to its tenacity, another disturbing aspect of WNV is its ability to travel. The U.S. public health community was stunned at the discovery of WNV in the United States in 1999 because it had previously been found only in Africa, the Middle East, and Europe.[13] Natural barriers are no longer sufficient to prevent the spread of disease because infected individuals can board airplanes and easily carry a disease across the world.

WNV provides an example of how important it is to have strong communication and coordination of information, not only between health care organizations and countries but also across professions, such as between public health professionals, physicians, veterinarians, and wildlife experts. Sharing information quickly can help make sure that decisions are made with the most current information. Practitioners who are familiar with the nuances of the disease will be more likely to spot it in patients and treat it early, thus lessening the symptoms.

SARS

SARS first emerged in China during the latter part of 2002.[14,15] There were unfortunate delays in recognizing the new illness, as well as in communicating about it with other countries. This was related to internal political and cultural decisions. SARS spread rapidly and, before the disease was contained, there were more than 8,000 probable cases of the virus in 29 countries. More than 10% of the victims died, with the case mortality rate reaching more than 50% for those over the age of 60.

One of the reasons that SARS spread so rapidly is the lack of detection capabilities in many countries and the lack of case reports to coordinating bodies such as the WHO. More than 100 countries do not have the laboratory expertise to spot even common diseases, so it is unlikely that they would spot a new virus until it had claimed many lives and spread to other countries.[16] Airline travel presents another opportunity to spread infection. Infected individuals can board an airplane and not only infect those people sitting around them, but can also carry the disease to another continent.

Communication breakdowns can also contribute to the spread of infection. Language and cultural barriers between nations can many times prevent prompt and clear disclosure of an emerging disease. Communication between health care organizations, as well as across national and international boundaries, offers the opportunity for early identification of infections, cooperation regarding border closings, and information sharing on the dynamics of an infection. For more information on the 2003 SARS outbreak and lessons learned from it, *see* Chapter 6.

Meningococcal Disease

Neisseria meningitidis is a leading cause of bacterial meningitis and other invasive bacterial infections both in the United States and worldwide. The WHO's conservative estimates for the meningococcal meningitis disease burden is 300,000 to 350,000 cases and more than 30,000 deaths each year.[17] All countries suffer from endemic meningococcal disease, which primarily affects children under 5 years of age.

In most of the developed world, meningococcal disease occurs at an endemic rate of 1–3 cases per 100,000 population per year. As many as half of these cases may be attributable to serogroup B, which is not preventable by the currently available vaccines. Among the other major serogroups, serogroup C is the most common cause of meningococcal disease.

In the developing world the disease pattern is markedly different. In sub-Saharan Africa, epidemic of serogroup A disease with rates of up to 1,000 to 2,000 cases per 100,000 population are of frequent occurrence. Recent outbreaks of serogroup W135 among pilgrims in Makkah and family contacts in their country of origin have caused major concern to Hajj (annual Islam pilgrimage to the foremost holy places) authorities in Saudi Arabia in the years 2000–2001. All pilgrims and at-risk local population must now be given quadrivalent polysaccharide meningococcal vaccine before performing the Hajj. That was effective in eliminating the problem in 2002.[18]

Diarrheal Disease

Diarrheal diseases remain a leading cause of preventable death, particularly among children under 5 in developing countries. Diarrhea is caused by infectious organisms, including viruses, bacteria, helminthes, and protozoa, that are transmitted through fecal-oral route. A strong relationship exists between poverty and an unhygienic environment and the incidence of diarrheal disease in developing countries. Poverty is associated with poor housing, overcrowding, and lack of access to clean water or sanitary disposal for fecal waste, all of which increase the frequency of diarrhea.[19]

Three to five billion episodes of watery diarrhea occur annually, with the highest incidence in children 6–24 months of age. Dehydration is the primary cause of mortality in children with diarrhea, and since the 1980s the annual mortality from diarrhea has come down from 6 million to 2 million cases. This is despite the fact that the median incidence of diarrheal disease in children under 5 in developing countries remains stable at around 3.2 to 3.5 episodes per child per year. This decline in mortality despite the lack of significant change in incidence is related to improved case management introduced in the early 1980s. By promoting the use of oral rehydration solution, exclusive breastfeeding, and personal and domestic hygiene, as well as increasing the protected water supply, existing interventions have been shown to be effective in reducing the burden of diarrheal disease in developing countries. The challenge ahead is to encourage the universal use of these interventions.[20]

Tuberculosis

Tuberculosis (TB) is the most common infectious disease worldwide, affecting one third of the global population and the leading cause of death from a curable infectious disease. The WHO estimated 8.8 million new cases in 2003, with 3.9 million cases of smear positive pulmonary TB and an estimated mortality of 1.7 million.[21] TB rates vary widely by region, with the highest rates in Africa (345 per 100,000 population annually) and the lowest rates in the Americas and Europe.

The rise of TB cases in Africa over the last decade is mainly a result of the burden of HIV infection, and in the former Soviet Union the increase is due to socioeconomic changes and decline of the health care system.[22] TB can be controlled by preventing infection, stopping progression from infection to active disease, and by treating the active disease.

Hepatitis

Hepatitis B (HBV) is the most common among the hepatitis viruses that cause chronic infection of the liver, with an estimated two billion people infected globally, 350 million of those suffering from chronic HBV infection. The patterns of HBV transmission vary considerably depending on the region of the world. In Western countries, HBV is acquired in adulthood, while in Asia and Africa the transmission is mostly in childhood, either from mother-to-child transmission or through contaminated needles and syringes. Prevention is possible through vaccination with the HBV vaccine.[23]

The global epidemiology of hepatitis C (HCV) is not as clear because most of the data the WHO uses to generate global estimates are from prevalence studies. The WHO estimates that there are at least 123 million people infected with HCV globally (2% of the world population). Countries in Africa and Asia have the highest incidence, while industrialized countries in North America and Europe have the lowest incidence. Risk factors frequently cited for disease transmission include transfusion of unscreened blood, injection drug use, and unsafe therapeutic injection. Because no vaccine is available to prevent the disease transmission, efforts should be focused on safer blood supply and safer injection practices in developing countries.[24]

Many other infectious diseases not discussed above (for example, typhoid, cholera, and dengue hemorrhagic fever) present ongoing challenges to populations in countries throughout the world and to the health care providers caring for those who are ill. Many people affected by these diseases must be cared for in health care organizations. Infection prevention and control efforts should minimize the risk of transmission of the infections during treatment and care.

Infection Clusters and Epidemics

The great majority of HAIs are endemic. They occur on an ongoing basis and require constant attention to ensure that they remain as low as possible. Methods to reduce or prevent endemic HAIs are described in Chapters 4 and 5.

Periodically, health care organizations experience clusters of infections and outbreaks of HAIs. Well-designed procedures and protocols are available to investigate these outbreaks in a systematic manner, determine the cause, and initiate interventions quickly.[25] System improvements and practices from one cluster or outbreak should prevent similar future outbreaks.

Organizations must have appropriate IPC procedures in place if an outbreak of an infectious disease occurs in the community that leads to patient admissions and the potential for transmission in the health care setting. During a crisis, there is insufficient time to educate health care professionals about the warning signs of certain diseases as well as the appropriate actions that they should take to prevent the transmission of these diseases. These challenges compel health care organizations to prepare in advance for an influx of infections from the community. This point was clearly illustrated in the SARS epidemic in Canada that lasted from February 2003 to August 2003. One of the most alarming aspects of the Canadian outbreak was the rapid spread of the disease among health care workers and between facilities. "We paid insufficient attention to maintaining and appropriately staffing hospital infection control teams and programs, and we paid dearly for this," comments Dr. Allison McGeer of Canada.[26] More about the SARS outbreak in Canada and the lessons learned appear in Chapter 6.

SARS had a devastating effect on patients, health care workers, and hospitals. It served as a wake-up call for the increased needs and requirements of IPC programs across all types of health care organizations.[27] No one knows when or if SARS will reappear, but similar diseases occur regularly. Health care organizations across the world should be vigilant and prepared for emerging or reemerging infectious diseases. When epidemics occur, organizations throughout the world must be prepared to respond rapidly and efficiently. Suggestions on how to do this appear in Chapters 4, 5, and 6.

Pandemics

Most infectious diseases do not become pandemics because it is more common for a microorganism to infect a relatively small number of people.[28] In some cases, an infectious disease can spread rapidly, jump continents, and affect large populations. If left unchecked, such a disease could become a pandemic. The severity of a pandemic depends on the organism's virulence, how rapidly it is able to spread from population to population, resistance or immunity of the population, and how effective prevention and response efforts are.[28] For example, in 1918 the Spanish influenza virus had a devastating impact. The strain was highly contagious and quite deadly. This pandemic killed more Americans than all the wars of the twentieth century[28] (*see* Sidebar 1-2).

Influenza

Health care has improved enormously since the influenza pandemic of 1918 and 1919 that caused an estimated 50 million deaths worldwide,[29] but that does not mitigate the possibility of catastrophic human loss in a modern-day pandemic. The U.S. Centers for Disease Control and Prevention (US CDC) estimates a pandemic could cause 2 million to 7.4 million human deaths globally, 134 million to 233 million outpatient

---

Sidebar 1-2

The Spanish Flu

The Spanish influenza pandemic was so severe that it is the catastrophe against which all other modern pandemics are measured. It is estimated that approximately 20% to 40% of the worldwide population became ill due to this virus and that approximately 50 million people died.[1] Between September 1918 and April 1919, approximately 500,000 deaths from the flu occurred in the United States alone. Many people died very quickly. Some who felt well in the morning became sick by noon and were dead by nightfall. Those infected who did not succumb to the disease within the first few days often died of complications such as pneumonia. One of the most unusual aspects of the Spanish flu was its ability to kill young, healthy adults. The attack rate and mortality of the disease was highest among adults 20 to 50 years old. The reasons for this remain uncertain but may be related to the activity of the immune system in healthy individuals. A virus of this severity has not been seen since,[2] but there is concern throughout the world that the current avian influenza A (H5N1) virus circulating in birds and other animals and causing disease in some humans may mutate to enable human-to-human transmission that could lead to a situation similar to the 1918 pandemic.

References

1. Taubenberger J.K.: 1918 influenza: The mother of all pandemics. *Emerg Infect Dis* 12(1):15–22, 2006.
2. National Vaccine Program Office: *Influenza Pandemics: How They Start, How They Spread, and Their Potential Impact.* U.S. Department of Health and Human Services. http://www.hhs.gov/nvpo/pandemics/flu2.htm (accessed Jun. 28, 2006).

---

visits, and 1.5 million to 5.2 million hospital admissions in high-income countries, and even greater human damage in low-income countries.[30]

Although relatively short in duration, influenza pandemics evolve quickly, take an immense toll, and leave social and economic problems in their wake. For example, an influenza pandemic could infect large numbers of health care professionals, and caring for those who are sick could become very difficult. If the majority of a community's police force is infected, it could become difficult to keep people safe. If air traffic controllers are all sick at once, air traffic could grind to a halt, stopping not only business and personal travel but, more important, the transport of life-saving vaccines and antiviral drugs.[28]

The threat of avian influenza, or "bird flu," is particularly significant at the time of this writing. Avian influenza viruses move quickly and brutally through poultry flocks—as quickly as within 48 hours—and have been found to infect humans in Azerbaijan, Cambodia, China, Djibouti, Egypt, Indonesia, Iraq, Thailand, Turkey, and Vietnam since 2003.[30] The more humans who are infected, combined with the proliferation of the virus among poultry and wild birds, boosts the probability that avian influenza could rise to the pandemic level[30] (*see* Sidebar 1-3).

HIV/AIDS

In 1982 public health officials began using the term *acquired immunodeficiency syndrome* (AIDS) to describe the occurrences of opportunistic infections in otherwise healthy people.[31] In 1985 the world acknowledged a global pandemic of HIV/AIDs.[32]

Initially, in the United States, AIDS was identified in gay men, and many people thought it occurred only in men who had sex with other men. Public fear, international distrust, and the unwillingness of the government to acknowledge a "gay" disease led to delays in identification and detection.[32] By 1982 transmission to women, injection drug users, hemophiliacs, and babies had been documented. Even then, it would be three more years before blood banks began screening blood for the presence of HIV. In 1985 the first transmission of the disease between a patient and a health care worker was reported.[32]

As more cases were identified, it became apparent that AIDS crosses cultural, social, and economic boundaries. The disease can occur in rich and poor, gay and straight, males and females, blacks and whites. According to UNAIDS/WHO (a joint program of the United Nations and World Health Organization), as of 2005, there were an estimated 38.6 million people worldwide living with AIDS.[33] Of those, an estimated 4.1 million were infected in 2005, and more than 2.8 million died of the virus.[33] Increasing proportions of worldwide AIDS patients are women. Though just under half of the world's AIDS sufferers are women, 59% of adults infected in sub-Saharan Africa are women, and 75% of persons age 15 to 24 living with HIV are female.[33]

Developing countries in particular are suffering from the pandemic and do not have access to the antiretroviral therapies needed to combat it. It is estimated that between 5 and 6 million adults in developing countries are currently in need of such therapies.[34]

Unsafe injection practices coupled with the unnecessary use of injections in low-income countries contribute to the burden of preventable blood-borne viral diseases, including HIV/AIDS.[35] The WHO estimates that 12 billion injections are given annually, with an estimated 160,000 HIV infections each year attributable to these practices.[36] Patients are at risk because single-use disposable and reusable needles and syringes are reused without adequate sterilization. Health care workers are also at risk because they are required to handle used injecting equipment in order to clean and sterilize it for use.

Injection safety can be improved by reducing the number of inappropriate injections given and by improving the sterility of the injection equipments used. The WHO in recent years recognized the link between unsafe injection practices in developing countries and the burden of blood-borne viral diseases. So in 1989 the WHO established the Safe

SIDEBAR 1-3

Infections That Know No Boundaries: Avian Influenza . . . The Next Great Pandemic?

Tim Uyeki, M.D., M.P.H., M.P.P., influenza expert, U.S. Centers for Disease Control and Prevention (US CDC), discusses human influenza and avian influenza A (H5N1) in Asia and elsewhere. This sidebar was adapted from Dr. Uyeki's presentation at the Joint Commission Resources/Association for Professionals in Infection Control and Epidemiology International Conference on Infections, 2005, San Francisco, California, USA. For more information on the Association for Professionals in Infection Control and Epidemiology, visit their Web site at http://www.apic.org. Note: Dr. Uyeki's data were current as of August 2005, and may or may not have changed. Please consult the Web sites of the US CDC (http://www.cdc.gov) or the World Health Organization (WHO) (http://www.who.int) for current data.

Influenza is not a new disease, but the reemergence of avian influenza A (H5N1) in 2003, and influenza vaccine shortages throughout the world have heightened awareness of the need for placing emphasis on pandemic planning.

Influenza is an acute respiratory illness. The etiology is infection with human influenza viruses that primarily infect epithelial cells of the upper respiratory tract that can replicate in the lower respiratory tract as well. The signs and symptoms of influenza differ by age of the patient.

The influenza viruses are dynamic; they continue to evolve. There are three types of influenza viruses that infect humans: types A, B, and C. Influenza B viruses do not cause pandemics, and type C viruses cause mild infections. Influenza A viruses—such as H1N1, H1N2, and H3N2—cause seasonal epidemics in the United States and worldwide. Novel influenza A viruses can cause global pandemics.

Influenza viruses have the propensity for genetic reassortment, which is the exchange of internal genes to create new viruses. These viruses continue to evolve through minor mutations through a process called "antigenic drift." This is what drives seasonal epidemics, and, therefore, global surveillance is essential year round, and worldwide. About 20% of children and 5% of adults worldwide develop symptomatic influenza A or B each year.[1]

The natural reservoir for new human influenza A virus subtypes is wild aquatic waterfowl: ducks or geese. All known influenza A viruses are found in these wild populations of waterfowl. H5N1 viruses are circulating among birds primarily in Asia, not among people. "Antigenic shift" results from the replacement of the hemagglutinin (HA) and sometimes the neuroaminidase with novel subtypes that have not been present in human viruses for a long time. The introduction of new HAs into human viruses usually results in a pandemic. Historically, this has resulted in widespread morbidity and mortality worldwide in all populations. Most people are aware of the 1918–1919 pandemic of the so-called Spanish flu, which was the emergence of H1N1 in humans and which caused an estimated 50 million deaths worldwide.[2] The 1957–1958 Asian flu, which was the emergence of H2N2 in humans, killed more than a million people worldwide. The H2N2 virus is no longer circulating in humans—it was replaced by H3N2, which emerged as the so-called

SIDEBAR 1-3—CONTINUED

Hong Kong flu in 1968–1969. There were an estimated 34,000 excess deaths in the United States.[3] That H3 came from an avian influenza A virus. It was a genetic reassortment between human and avian influenza A viruses. H3N2 viruses continue to circulate worldwide causing tremendous morbidity and mortality.

Are we going to have an influenza pandemic? I believe we will. I don't know if it's going to be H5N1, and I don't know when it's going to be. Since 2003 there has been an unprecedented, widespread outbreak of highly pathogenic H5N1 viruses among poultry. The majority of poultry infected are probably in what we call "backyard flocks," not commercial poultry farms. More than 160 million poultry have died or have been killed. H5N1 is now endemic in poultry in many countries throughout the world, including Vietnam, Thailand, Laos, Cambodia, Indonesia, Malaysia, China, and, more recently, Russia, Kazakhstan, Turkey, Egypt, and Jordan. The list is expanding rapidly.[4]

Probable limited person-to-person transmission of H5N1 virus is not new. What is the risk of H5N1 for health care workers? One study from Vietnam reviewed human-to-human transmission of influenza A H5N1 in hospital employees by testing health care workers exposed to confirmed and probable patients with the infection. None of the health care workers had detectable antibodies to the virus.[5] Their data suggest that H5N1 viruses were not readily transmitted from person to person during this study. But all you can conclude from these findings is that they apply to those specific situations at that time, because these viruses are continuing to evolve.

The WHO published interim infection prevention and control recommendations for suspected H5N1 patients in 2004 and updated them in February 2006.[4] Full barrier precautions, which include standard, contact, and airborne precautions (plus eye protection), should be used when possible when providing care for suspected or confirmed avian influenza patients with close patient contact and during aerosol generating procedures. Because some elements of full barrier precautions (particularly airborne precautions) may not be available in all health care facilities, minimal requirements for caring for H5N1 patients should include standard, contact, and droplet precautions. We also recommend annual influenza vaccinations for health care workers. It's not going help protect against H5N1, but it could potentially reduce the risk of coinfection with H5N1 and human influenza A viruses and then decrease the risk of reassortment. And what's really important is active surveillance of health care workers who have had contact with H5N1 patients.

There is no currently available human H5N1 vaccine. Phase I and II human clinical trials of a monovalent, inactivated H5N1 vaccine are going on right now in the United States. Other countries are planning research to look at adjuvant vaccines, and other dose-sparing strategies are being examined, such as intradermal vaccine administration. Researchers in Vietnam have developed an inactivated H5N1 vaccine that they have tried in animals and plan to try in humans. Antiviral stockpiling has also received a lot of attention, with a focus on the drug Oseltamivir. Many countries are planning to stockpile Oseltamivir, which means that there will be global competition for the drug.

(continued)

SIDEBAR 1-3—CONTINUED

The good news is that there's no evidence of sustained human-to-human transmission of H5N1 viruses and no pandemic now. However, the H5N1 virus is endemic in poultry and cannot be eradicated soon. These viruses are evolving. Human influenza A viruses are circulating among people in many countries. Thus, there's the risk of coinfection and genetic reassortment.

Very severe human disease has occurred with H5N1 virus infection, and the real key to reducing the public health threat of a pandemic is to control this problem in poultry. Clearly, a lot of international coordination, assistance, and planning is needed on the national, regional, and global levels, and health care organizations everywhere must prepare for the possibility of a catastrophic pandemic.

References

1. Nicholson K.G., Wood J.M., Zamboon M.: Influenza. *Lancet* 362:1733–1745, Nov. 2003.
2. Johnson N.P., Mueller J.: Updating the accounts: Global mortality of the 1918–1920 "Spanish" influenza pandemic. *Bull Hist Med* 76:105–115, Spring 2002.
3. Peters C.J.: Hurrying toward disaster? *Perspectives in Health Magazine* 7, 2002. Pan American Health Organization. http://www.paho.org/English/DPI/Number14_article3_2.htm (accessed Jun. 28, 2006).
4. World Health Organization: *Avian Influenza ("Bird Flu") and the Significance of Its Transmission to Humans.* http://www.who.int/mediacentre/factsheets/avian_influenza/en/ (accessed Jun. 28, 2006).
5. Liem N.T., Lim W.: World Health Organization International Avian Influenza Investigation Team, Vietnam. Lack of H5N1 avian influenza transmission to hospital employees, Hanoi, 2004. *Emerg Infect Dis* 11:210–215, Feb. 2005.

Injection Global Network, which is an international alliance of all organizations concerned with achieving safer use of injections globally.[37]

Because there is no known cure for HIV/AIDS, the probability that it will continue to infect individuals is high. Risky behavior such as unprotected sex still occurs, so individuals can still transmit it. Certain populations such as the poor and the uninsured cannot afford AIDS therapy and thus will continue to die from it. Because of all this, health care organizations must continue to address the issues surrounding AIDS.

Increased HIV testing helps get a handle on the volume of the disease, identify the populations that are being affected by it, determine the behaviors that are transmitting it, and direct prevention efforts. Early warning signs of resurgence can be tracked through this data collection, and the spread of the infection to a new population can be identified.[38]

Bioterrorism

The idea that biological weapons can and will be used in an act of terror against nations and people has become more than just the worry of a select few. Releases of biological agents or materials (or threats of releases) as weapons of mass destruction have the potential to evoke human injury and destruction, as well as widespread public fear and panic.[39]

The health care community in each country must work closely with public health officials, law enforcement, and the military to ensure public safety in the face of bioterrorism threats. A recent study indicated that nearly 75% of U.S. IPC professionals surveyed believed a terrorist attack with biological agents is likely to occur in the United States sometime in the next five years. However, only one third of those individuals believed that their community would be at risk.[40] This statistic is worrisome because a bioterrorism event could affect all types of health care organizations of varying sizes in communities around the world.

A significant challenge in preparing for a potential bioterrorism event is anticipating the nature of the event and predicting what IPC issues will come up. The type of organism, the location of the release, the composition of the infected population, and the use of health care organizations by infected people to get treatment will all affect how the specific events of a bioterrorist act unfold. Although there are a multitude of potential bioterrorism agents, following is a brief discussion of two that have received increased media attention in the United States during the past few years.

Anthrax

Anthrax is not spread through direct person-to-person contact. Rather, the disease is contracted through direct exposure to *Bacillus anthracis* spores.[41] Most likely, in a bioterrorism event, only the individuals coming in contact with spores would be affected. However, placement of spores in a large air-conditioning unit that could distribute them across a wide space could prove catastrophic if early identification and rapid response do not occur.

If untreated, anthrax can lead to septicemia, meningitis, and death. In persons exposed to anthrax, infection can be prevented with antibiotic treatment, and early antibiotic treatment can also help enhance a person's chance of survival.[41] Early identification of an anthrax attack would lead to rapid antibiotic distribution and containment, so national and local surveillance activities are needed to help mitigate the effects of a possible attack.

Smallpox

Smallpox is transmitted through direct and fairly prolonged face-to-face contact. In addition, an individual can also be infected through direct contact with infected bodily fluids or contaminated objects such as bedding and clothing.[42] In many ways, the threat of smallpox as a biological weapon is more serious than anthrax. Because it can spread with person-to-person contact, terrorists can infect themselves with the virus and then travel to multiple countries, using their bodies to spread the infection in public areas. The scope of such an event would be enormous.[16] Multiple countries could be affected. These nations would need to work together to put an end to the infection.

There is no specific treatment for smallpox, and the only prevention is vaccination. In fact, a worldwide vaccination program that started in the 1950s has all but eradicated the disease. Some supplies of the virus still exist, which has caused some concern that the disease will be used as a weapon in a terrorist event.[42] Because the disease has been eliminated in many parts of the world, routine vaccination no longer occurs. People who received the smallpox vaccine prior to 1980 probably have little to no immunity to smallpox today and in the case of an epidemic would require vaccination.[42] Should a bioterrorism event involving smallpox occur, infected patients would need to be identified and isolated. Health care workers tending to these individuals would need to be vaccinated before they could provide services. Transmission would need to be reduced through the vaccination of close contacts of the isolating cases. Depending on the nature of the attack, a large-scale vaccination might be necessary, in which case public health organizations and other health care organizations such as ambulatory clinics would have to cope with the logistics of vaccinating the entire community.

Although both anthrax and smallpox have the potential to wreak havoc across the world, health care organizations can arm themselves to effectively respond to outbreaks, as well as proactively address dangerous situations. Organizations should develop response plans that can be activated in the event of a bioterrorist act. Communication between health care organizations, states, and countries is crucial to identify threats early and address issues rapidly to preserve the safety of patients. Suggestions on how to facilitate communication and prompt response to a biological emergency appear in Chapter 5.

Joint Commission International's Response to the IPC Crisis

The progressively changing area of IPC and the concerns associated with it have led JCI to examine its leadership role with health care organizations worldwide.

The JCI infection prevention and control standards—Prevention and Control of Infections (PCI)—require health care organizations to identify and reduce the risks of acquiring and transmitting infections among patients, staff, practitioners, and visitors. The standards cover both direct patient care activities and those used to support patient care. The new standards emphasize several areas of IPC, including the following:
- Leadership involvement
- Surveillance
- Ongoing risk assessment
- Appropriate staffing
- Effectiveness monitoring

An in-depth look at the current PCI standards appears in Chapter 2.

Other Initiatives to Address the IPC Crisis

Joint Commission International holds IPC as a priority, and organizations such as the WHO and the US CDC have contributed guidelines and expertise toward the reduction of infections. Following are brief discussions of some of the initiatives from JCI, the WHO, the US CDC, and the Institute for Healthcare Improvement (IHI) that are designed to help organizations address the issues surrounding IPC to improve patient safety and quality of care.

International Patient Safety Goals

In addition to its PCI standards, the Joint Commission has incorporated the issue of IPC into its International Patient Safety Goals (ISPGs). The applicable goal states that all organizations must "comply with current published and generally accepted hand hygiene guidelines," noting that "not all countries have a CDC (Centers for Disease Control and Prevention) or may not recognize the US CDC."[43] Starting 1 January 2007, the IPSGs will be an official part of the JCI accreditation decision process.

Joint Commission Resources' International Conferences on IPC

In September 2005 Joint Commission Resources, in tandem with Joint Commission International and the Association for Professionals in Infection Control and Epidemiology (APIC), sponsored "Think Globally, Act Locally: An International Conference on Infections That Have No Boundaries" in San Francisco, California, USA. Nearly 200 participants—ranging from IPC professionals and nurse managers to emergency planners and students—delved into the state of IPC and gained understanding as to how quickly emerging and reemerging pathogens can spread and drafted recommendations regarding what should be done at the global, local, and organizational level to help prevent, identify, and control their spread. In August 2006 the same organizations presented a joint conference to examine health care–associated and community-associated methicillin-resistant *Staphylococcus aureus* (MRSA), another worldwide infection problem.

The WHO and the Joint Commission International Center for Patient Safety

On 13 October 2005, the WHO launched its "Global Patient Safety Challenge: Clean Care Is Safer Care" in Geneva, Switzerland, and published its *WHO Guidelines on Hand Hygiene in Health Care* (Advanced Draft). Highlights of the WHO hand hygiene guidelines appear in Chapter 2, and the complete document can be downloaded at http://www.who.int/ patientsafety/information_centre/who_ghhhcad/en/index.html. A final version of the document will be issued in 2007. The Joint Commission International Center for Patient Safety (http://www.jcipatientsafety.org) strongly supports this and other projects to reduce health care–associated infections. The Center's Patient Safety Practices resource center (http://www.jcipatientsafety.org/show.asp?durki=11787) includes a wealth of information on hand hygiene and infection prevention and control.

U.S. Centers for Disease Control and Prevention Programs

The US CDC boasts a number of programs and publications targeting hand hygiene, including the following:

- *Clean Hands Save Lives!* campaign—why and how to clean hands, including instructions for hand hygiene in emergency situations (*see* http://www.cdc.gov/cleanhands/)
- *The Clean Hands Coalition*—an alliance of public and private partners creating initiatives to improve health and save lives through clean hands
- *Guideline for Hand Hygiene in Health-Care Settings*—a comprehensive 62-page publication (2002; available online at http://www.cdc.gov/handhygiene/) featuring recommendations of the Healthcare Infection Control Practices Advisory Committee (HICPAC) in partnership with the Society for Healthcare Epidemiology of America (SHEA), the Association of Professionals in Infection Control and Epidemiology (APIC), and the Infectious Disease Society of America (IDSA)

Institute for Healthcare Improvement's Hand Hygiene Tool

The IHI has collaborated with the US CDC, APIC, and SHEA to produce *How-to Guide: Improving Hand Hygiene*, a 32-page toolkit that includes tips, forms, and current information for staff members looking to enhance their hand hygiene practices. The toolkit is included in this book as Appendix 2, starting on page 169.

Conclusion

Infection prevention and control are critical components of safe, high-quality care. Those organizations that embrace the concepts of infection prevention and control and implement systems to identify, address, and prevent the spread of infections help create a culture based on safety and an organization rooted in quality. To create such a culture, organizations must continually examine, evaluate, and act on IPC issues and view IPC from a perspective that places the health and safety of patients as the first priority.

References

1. World Health Organization: *Blood Safety and Clinical Technology Guidelines on Prevention and Control of Hospital Associated Infections.* http://w3.whosea.org/en/Section10/Section17/Section53/Section362_1107.htm (accessed Jun. 28, 2006).
2. Vincent J.L.: Nosocomial infections in adult intensive-care units. *Lancet* 361:2068–2077, Jun. 2003.
3. Starfield B.: Is US health really the best in the world? *JAMA* 284:483–485, Jul. 2000.
4. National Audit Office: *Improving Patient Care by Reducing the Risk of Hospital Acquired Infection: A Progress Report.* London: Stationery Office, 2004.
5. Ponce de Leon-Rosales, S.P., et al.: Prevalence of infection in intensive care units in Mexico: A multicenter study. *Crit Care Med* 28:1316–1321, May 2000.
6. Zaidi A.K., et al.: Hospital-acquired neonatal infections in developing countries. *Lancet* 365:1175–1188, Mar. 2005.
7. McDonald L.C., et al.: SARS in healthcare facilities, Toronto and Taiwan. *Emerg Infect Dis* 10:777–781, May 2004.
8. Seto W.H., et al.: Effectiveness of precautions against droplets and contact in prevention of nosocomial transmission of severe acute respiratory syndrome (SARS). *Lancet* 361:1519–1520, May 2003.
9. O'Leary D.: Opening comments at the Joint Commission's Infection Control Conference, Chicago, Nov. 17, 2003.
10. Levy E., Fischetti M.: *The New Killer Diseases.* New York: Crown Publishers, 2003.
11. National Advisory Committee on SARS and Public Health: *Learning from SARS.* Ottawa, ON: Health Canada, Oct. 2003.
12. Centers for Disease Control and Prevention: *West Nile Virus.* http://www.cdc.gov/ncidod/dvbid/westnile/background.htm (accessed Jun. 28, 2006).
13. Trust for America's Health: *Animal-Borne Epidemics Out of Control: Threatening the Nation's Health.* Aug. 2003. http://www.pewtrusts.com/pdf/tfah_animal_borne_080503.pdf (accessed Jun. 28, 2006).
14. Christian M.D., et al.: Severe acute respiratory syndrome. *Clin Infect Dis* 38:1420–1427, May 15, 2004.
15. Poutanen S.M., Low D.E.: Severe acute respiratory syndrome: An update. *Curr Opin Infect Dis* 17:287–294, Aug. 2004.
16. Vedantam S.: WHO assails wealthy nations on bioterror. *Washington Post,* Nov. 5, 2003.
17. Memish Z.A.: Meningococcal disease and travel. *Clin Infect Dis* 34:84–90, Jan. 2002.
18. Ahmed Q.A., Arabi Y.M., Memish Z.A.: Health risks at the Hajj. *Lancet* 367:1008–1015, Mar. 2006.
19. Fewtrell L., Colford J.M. Jr.: Water, sanitation and hygiene in developing countries: Interventions and diarrhea—A review. *Water Sci Technol* 52(8):133–142, 2005.
20. O'Ryan M., Prado V., Pickering L.K.: A millennium update on pediatric diarrheal illness in the developing world. *Semin Pediatr Infect Dis* 16:125–136, Apr. 2005.

21. Dye, C.: Global epidemiology of tuberculosis. *Lancet* 367:938–940, Mar. 2006.

22. Corbett E.L., et al.: The growing burden of tuberculosis: Global trends and interactions with the HIV epidemic. *Arch Int Med* 163:1009–1021, May 2003.

23. Lavanchy D.: Worldwide epidemiology of HBV infection, disease burden, and vaccine prevention. *J Clin Viro* 34 (suppl. 1):S1–S3, Dec. 2005.

24. Shepard C.W., Finelli L., Alter M.J.: Global epidemiology of hepatitis C virus infection. *Lancet Infect Dis* 5:558–567, Sep. 2005.

25. Checko, P.J.: Outbreak investigation. In Pfeiffer J. (ed.): *APIC Text of Infection Control and Epidemiology.* Washington, D.C.: Association for Professionals in Infection Control and Epidemiology, Inc., 2000, pp. 15-1–15-9.

26. CDC SARS Meeting. Sep. 12, 2003, Atlanta, Georgia.

27. Loutfy M.R., et al.: Hospital preparedness and SARS. *Emerg Infect Dis* 10:771–776, May 2005.

28. National Vaccine Program Office. *Influenza Pandemics: How They Start, How They Spread, and Their Potential Impact.* U.S. Department of Health and Human Services. http://www.hhs.gov/nvpo/pandemics/flu2.htm (accessed Jun. 28, 2006).

29. Taubenberger J.K.: 1918 influenza: The mother of all pandemics. *Emerg Infect Dis* 12(1):15–22, 2006.

30. World Health Organization (WHO): *Cumulative Number of Confirmed Human Cases of Avian Influenza A/(H5N1) Reported to WHO.* http://www.who.int/csr/disease/avian_influenza/en/ (accessed Jun. 28, 2006).

31. Centers for Disease Control and Prevention. *HIV/AIDS.* http://www.cdc.gov/hiv/ (accessed Jun. 28, 2006).

32. Berg D.: Impact of infections on communities and health care organizations: Lessons learned. Paper presented at the Joint Commission on Accreditation of Healthcare Organization's Infection Control Conference, Chicago, Nov. 17, 2003.

33. UNAIDS: *2006 Report on the Global AIDS Epidemic.* http://www.unaids.org/en/HIV_data/2006GlobalReport/default.asp (accessed Jun. 28, 2006).

34. World Health Organization: *International Treatment Access Coalition (ITAC).* http://www.who.int/hiv/itac/en/ (accessed Jun. 28, 2006).

35. Hauri A.M., Armstrong G.L., Hutin Y.J.: The global burden of disease attributable to contaminated injections given in health care settings. *Int J STD AIDS* 15:7–16, Jan. 2004.

36. Kermode M.: Healthcare worker safety is a pre-requisite for injection safety in developing countries. *Int J Inf Dis* 8:325–327, Nov. 2004.

37. Kermode M.: Unsafe injections in low income country health settings: Need for injection safety promotion to prevent the spread of blood borne viruses. *Health Promot Int* 19:95–103, Mar. 2004.

38. Karon J., et al.: HIV in the United States at the turn of the century: An epidemic in transition. *Am J Public Health* 91:1060–1068, Jul. 2001.

39. World Health Organization: *Preparedness for Deliberate Epidemics: Programme of Work for the Biennium 2004–2005.* http://www.who.int/csr/resources/publications/deliberate/WHO_CDS_CSR_LYO_2004_8.pdf (accessed Jun. 28, 2006).

40. Shadel B., et al.: Infection control practitioners' perceptions and educational needs regarding bioterrorism: Results from a national needs assessment survey. *Am J Infect Control* 31:129–134, May 2003.

41. Centers for Disease Control and Prevention. *Anthrax.* http://www.cdc.gov/nip/diseases/anthrax/default.htm (accessed Jun. 28, 2006).
42. Centers for Disease Control and Prevention. *Smallpox.* http://www.bt.cdc.gov/agent/smallpox (accessed Jun. 28, 2006).
43. Joint Commission International Center for Patient Safety: *International Patient Safety Goals.* http://www.jcipatientsafety.org/show.asp?durki=11753&site=164&return=93 35 (accessed Jun. 28, 2006).

Further Readings

Ducel G., Gabry J., Nicolle L.: *Prevention of Hospital-Acquired Infections: A Practical Guide.* Geneva: World Health Organization, 2002.
Huskins W.C., et al.: Infection control in countries with limited resources. In Mayhall G. (ed.): *Hospital Epidemiology and Infection Control,* 3rd ed. Philadelphia: Lippincott Williams & Wilkins, 2004, pp. 1889–1921.
Joint Commission Resources: *Infection Control Issues in the Environment of Care.* Oakbrook Terrace, IL: Joint Commission on Accreditation of Healthcare Organizations, 2005.
Mayhall C.G.: *Hospital Epidemiology and Infection Control,* 4th ed. Baltimore: Williams & Wilkins, 2004.
Pittet D., Donaldson L.: Clean care is safer care: A worldwide priority. *Lancet* 366:1246–1247, Oct. 8, 2005.
Soule B., Memish Z.: Infection control practice: Global preparedness for future challenges. *J Chemother* 13 (suppl. 1):45–49, Apr. 2001.

Resources

The following readings were gathered for use in *Information Resources in Infection Control,* Fourth Edition (Editor: Nizam Damani M.D., MBBS, MSc, FRCPI, FRCPath), due in 2006 from the International Federation of Infection Control (IFIC). The full document will be available online at IFIC's Web site: http://www.theific.org/publications.asp. NOTE: Some of these resources may appear at the end of more than one chapter, due to their applicability to more than one aspect of infection prevention and control.

American Thoracic Society; Centers for Disease Control and Prevention; Infectious Diseases Society of America: Controlling tuberculosis in the United States: Recommendations from the American Thoracic Society, CDC, and the Infectious Diseases Society of America. *Am J Respir Crit Care Med* 172:1169–1227, Nov. 2005.

Association for Professionals in Infection Control and Epidemiology, Inc.: Responsibility for interpretation of the PPD tuberculin skin test. *Am J Infect Control* 27(1):56–58, 1999.

Association for Professionals in Infection Control and Epidemiology, Inc./Society for Healthcare Epidemiology of America: Requirements for infrastructure and essential activities of infection control and epidemiology in hospitals: A consensus panel report. *Infect Control Hosp Epidemiol* 19:114–124, Feb. 1998. http://www.shea-online.org/publications/shea_position_papers.cfm.

Association of Anaesthetists of Great Britain and Ireland: *Infection Control in Anaesthesia.* 2002. http://www.aagbi.org.uk/.

Australian Department of Health and Ageing: *Infection Control Guidelines for the Prevention of Transmission of Infectious Diseases in the Health Care Setting.* 2004. http://www.health.gov.au/internet/wcms/publishing.nsf/ Content/icg-guidelines-index.htm-copy6.

British Medical Association: *Healthcare Associated Infections: A Guide for Healthcare Professionals.* London: BMA Publishing, 2006.

Centers for Disease Control and Prevention: Guidelines for preventing the transmission of *Mycobacterium tuberculosis* in health-care settings, 2005. *MMWR Recomm Rep* 54:1–141, Dec. 30, 2005. http://www.cdc.gov/mmwr/PDF/rr/rr5417.pdf.

———: Control and prevention of meningococcal disease and control and prevention of serogroup C meningococcal disease: Evaluation and management of suspected outbreaks. *MMWR Recomm Rep* 46:1–22, Feb. 14, 1997. http://www.cdc.gov/mmwr/PDF/rr/rr4605.pdf.

———: CDC definitions of surgical sites infections, 1992: A modification of the CDC definitions of wound infections. *Am J Infect Control* 20:271–274, Oct. 1992.

————: CDC definitions for nosocomial infections, 1988. *Am J Infect Control* 16:128–140, Jun. 1988.

Department of Health Hospital Infection Working Group and Public Health Laboratory Service: *Hospital Infection Control: Guidance on the Control of Infection in Hospitals (The Cooke Report).* London: Department of Health, 1995.

Department of Health (UK): The *epic* Project: Developing national evidence-based guidelines for preventing healthcare associated infections. *J Hosp Infect* 47 (suppl.):S1–S82, Jan. 2001. http://www.dh.gov.uk/assetRoot/04/07/73/68/04077368.PDF.

————:*The Prevention and Control of Tuberculosis in the United Kingdom: Tuberculosis and Homeless People.* London: Department of Health, 1996.

Department of Health (UK) and Public Health Medicine Environmental Group: *Guidelines on the Control of Infection in Residential and Nursing Homes.* London: Department of Health, 1996.

Embry F.C., Chinnes L.F.: Draft definitions for surveillance of infections in home health care. *Am J Infect Control* 28:449–453, Dec. 2000.

French G., Friedman C. (eds.): *Infection Control: Basic Concepts and Practices, 2nd ed.* International Federation of Infection Control. 2003. http://www.theific.org/oldsite/Manual/toc.htm.

Harries A.D., Maher D., Nunn P.: Practical and affordable measures for the protection of health care workers from tuberculosis in low-income countries. *Bull World Health Organ* 75(5):477–489, 1997.

Health Canada, Laboratory Centre for Disease Control: Infection control guidelines: Routine practices and additional precautions for preventing the transmission of infection in health care. *Canada Communicable Disease Report* 25 (suppl. 4):1–155, Jul. 1999. http://www.phac-aspc.gc.ca/publi-cat/ccdr-rmtc/99pdf/cdr25s4e.pdf.

Horan T.C., Gaynes R.P.: Surveillance of nosocomial infections. In Mayall, C.G., Ed., *Hospital Epidemiology and Infection Control*, 3rd ed., Philadelphia: Lippincott Williams & Wilkins, 2004: pp. 1659–1702.

Infectious Disease Society of America and the Centers for Disease Control and Prevention: Practice guidelines for the treatment of tuberculosis. *Clin Infect Dis* 31:633–699, Oct. 2000.

Masterton R., Teare L., Richards J.: Hospital Infection Society/Association of Medical Microbiologists "Towards a Consensus II" Workshop I hospital-acquired infection and risk management. *J Hosp Infect* 51:17–20, May 2002.

McKibben L.: Guidance on public reporting of healthcare–associated infections: Recommendations of the Healthcare Infection Control Practices Advisory Committee. *Infect Control Hospl Epidemiol* 26(6):580–587, 2005.

National Audit Office (UK): *The Challenge of Hospital Acquired Infection.* London: Stationery Office, 2001.

————: *The Management and Control of Hospital Acquired Infection in Acute NHS Trusts in England.* London: Stationery Office, 2000.

National Collaborating Centre for Chronic Conditions: *Tuberculosis: Clinical Diagnosis and Management of Tuberculosis, and Measures for Its Prevention and Control.* London: Royal College of Physicians, 2006. http://www.rcplondon.ac.uk/pubs/books/TB/Tuberculosis2.pdf.

National Institute for Clinical Excellence: Prevention of healthcare-associated infection in primary care and community care. *J Hospl Infect* 55 (suppl. 2): S1–S127, Jun. 2004. http://www.nice.org.uk/pdf/Infection_control_fullguideline.pdf.

Office of Health Economics (UK): *Hospital Acquired Infection.* London: Office of Health Economics, 1997.

Plowman R.P., et al.: *The Socioeconomic Burden of Hospital Acquired Infection.* London: Public Health Laboratory Service, 1999.

Public Health Agency of Canada: Guidelines for preventing the transmission of tuberculosis in Canadian health care facilities and other institutional settings. *Canada Communicable Disease Report* 22S1, Apr. 1996. http://www.phac-aspc.gc.ca/publicat/ccdr-rmtc/96vol22/22s1/index.html.

Public Health Laboratory Service (PHLS): *Preventing Hospital Acquired Infection: Clinical Guidelines.* London: PHLS, 1997.

Public Health Laboratory Service, Public Health Medicine Environmental Group, Scottish Centre for Infection and Environmental Health: Guidelines for public health management of meningococcal disease in the UK. *Communicable Disease and Public Health* 5(3):187–204, 2002.

Scottish Department of Health: *The Control of Tuberculosis in Scotland.* Scottish Office Department of Health, 1998.

————: *Scottish Infection Manual: Guidance on Core Standards for the Control of Infection in Hospitals, Health Care Premises and the Community Interface.* Edinburgh: Scottish Executive, 1998.

Scottish Executive, NHS Scotland: *Infection Control Standards for Adult Care Homes: Final Standards.* Edinburgh: Scottish Executive, Mar. 2005. http://www.scotland.gov.uk/Publications/2005/03/19927/42762.

Society for Cardiovascular Angiography and Interventions: Infection control guidelines for the cardiac catheterization laboratory: Society guidelines revisited. *Catheter Cardiovasc Interv* 67:78–86, Jan 2006.

World Health Organization (WHO): *Practical Guidelines for Infection Control in Healthcare Facilities.* New Delhi: WHO, 2004. http://www.wpro.who.int/NR/rdonlyres/006EF250-6B11-42B4-BA17-C98D413BE8B8/0/Final_guidelines_Dec2004.pdf.

————: *Guidelines on Prevention and Control of Hospital Associated Infections.* New Delhi: WHO, 2002.

————: *Prevention of Hospital Acquired Infections: A Practical Guide.* 2nd ed. Geneva: WHO, 2002.
http://whqlibdoc.who.int/hq/2002/WHO_CDS_CSR_EPH_2002.12.pdf.

————: *Tuberculosis Handbook.* Geneva: WHO, 2000.

————: *Guidelines for the Management of Drug-Resistant Tuberculosis.* Geneva: WHO, 1997.

Joint Commission International's Infection Prevention and Control Standards and Requirements
A Detailed Study

The prevention and control of infections represent one of the most significant safety initiatives for a health care organization. Infections can be acquired in any health care setting, transferred between organizations, or brought in from the community. Because infections are a significant safety risk for patients and other care recipients and for health care workers, infection prevention and control (IPC) must be high on every organization's list of priorities.

To help organizations focus on IPC issues and address related challenges, Joint Commission International (JCI) has developed the Prevention and Control of Infections (PCI) standards in the hospital, ambulatory care, and care continuum accreditation manuals (*see* Appendix 1, "JCI Prevention and Control of Infections Standards and Compliance Checklist"). IPC issues are also covered in the "Quality Management and Improvement System" (QMS) chapter of the clinical laboratories manual, as well as in the "Quality Management and Improvement" (QMI) and the "Exposure to and Transmission of Biologic and Chemical Agents" (BCA) chapters of the medical transport manual (*see* Box 2-2 on page 30). In addition to the standards, JCI has introduced for 2006 an International Patient Safety Goal related to IPC that requires organizations to comply with the hand hygiene guidelines of the World Health Organization (WHO) (or other appropriate local agency).

The purpose of this chapter is to provide an in-depth look at the standards and the International Patient Safety Goal to help organizations understand the requirements of Joint Commission International regarding PCI. There is a compliance checklist in Appendix 1. The list of PCI standards only is provided in Box 2-1, and strategies for standards compliance are covered in depth in Chapters 4 and 5.

Box 2-1

JCI Infection Prevention and Control (PCI) Standards

The following is a list of all standards for the PCI chapter in the *Joint Commission International Accreditation Standards for Hospitals* (Second Edition) and the *Joint Commission International Accreditation Standards for Ambulatory Care*. Asterisks (*) denote standards applicable to JCI's care continuum accreditation program; standards preceded by an asterisk and dagger (*†) are applicable in care continuum, but not to home care. The standards printed in **bold** typeface are core standards that all organizations must meet to be accredited. These standards are effective as of the date of this publication (October 2006), but hospital standards will be updated in 2007.

*PCI.1 The organization designs and implements a coordinated program to reduce the risks of nosocomial infections in patients and health care workers.

*PCI.1.1 All patient, staff, and visitor areas of the organization are included in the infection control program.

***PCI.2 The organization establishes the focus of the nosocomial infection prevention and reduction program.**

***PCI.3 The organization identifies the procedures and processes associated with the risk of infection and implements strategies to reduce infection risk.**

***PCI.4 Gloves, masks, soap, and disinfectants are available and used correctly when required.**

*†PCI.5 Cultures are routinely obtained from designated sites in the organization associated with significant infection risk.

PCI.6 One or more individuals oversee all infection control activities. This individual(s) is qualified in infection control practices through education, training, experience, or certification.

***PCI.7 A designated individual or group monitors and coordinates infection control activities in the organization.**

PCI.8 Coordination of infection control activities involves medicine, nursing, and others as appropriate to the organization.

BOX 2-1—CONTINUED

***PCI.9** The infection control program is based on current scientific knowledge, accepted practice guidelines, and applicable law and regulation.

PCI.10 Organization information management systems support the infection control program.

PCI.11 The infection control process is integrated with the organization's overall program for quality improvement and patient safety.

PCI.11.1 The organization tracks infection risks, infection rates, and trends in nosocomial infections.

PCI.11.2 Monitoring includes using indicators related to infection issues that are epidemiologically important to the organization.

***PCI.11.3** The organization uses risk, rate, and trend information to design or modify processes to reduce nosocomial infections to the lowest possible levels.

PCI.11.4 The organization compares its infection control rates with other organizations through comparative databases.

***†PCI.11.5** The results of infection monitoring in the organization are regularly communicated to staff, doctors, and management.

PCI.11.6 The organization reports information on infections to appropriate external public health agencies.

***PCI.12** The organization provides education on infection control practices to staff, doctors, patients, and, as appropriate, family and other caregivers.

PCI.12.1 All staff receives an orientation to the organization's infection control policies and practices.

PCI.12.2 All staff is educated in infection control when new policies are implemented and when significant trends are noted in surveillance data.

The PCI Standards

The JCI standards were created to respond to requests from the international community for external, objective, standards-based evaluation of health care practices and organizations. The goal of the accreditation program is to stimulate demonstration of continuous, sustained improvement in health care organizations by applying international consensus standards and indicators. The PCI standards require a focused look at IPC across an organization and have an underlying philosophy of quality management, continuous quality improvement, and patient safety. These standards guide

Box 2-2

Nonhospital Infection
Prevention and Control–Related Standards

Clinical Laboratories

Quality Management and Improvement System (QMS)

QMS.7.2.2 Policies and procedures define laboratory safety procedures and controls and how environmental requirements are supported and maintained.

Medical Transport

Quality Management and Improvement (QMI)

QMI.3.7 Monitoring includes surveillance and reporting of infections, biologic and hazardous materials control, environmental and practice issues.

Exposure to and Transmission of Biologic and Chemical Agents (BCA)

BCA.1 The organization designs and implements a coordinated program to reduce the risks of infections.

the organization leadership to establish and maintain a comprehensive, integrated IPC program that is adequately supported and well managed.

The standards discuss the components of a comprehensive IPC program and the resources and support systems necessary to successfully implement such a program. There are three parts to the PCI standards: the standard, intent, and measurable element(s).

The Standard

The 12 PCI standards define the performance expectation, structures, or functions that must be in place for IPC. These standards were developed using a consensus process with a task force of international experts. They are based on accreditation experiences during recent years in more than 30 countries. The standards are validated through accreditation surveys and are designed to incorporate local or national laws and regulations. JCI has determined that organizations being surveyed must satisfactorily meet the requirements of selected "core" standards for the prevention and control of infection to achieve accreditation. The core standards are designed to create a culture of patient safety and lead organizations to best practice levels to protect fundamental patient and family rights, reduce risks during patient care processes, and enhance a safe environment where care is provided. The 7 core PCI standards are PCI.2, .3, .4, .6, .7, .8, and .11 and are indicated by bold printing in the list of standards. The other 5 standards (PCI.1, .5, .9,

.10, and .12), although considered "non-core," are still important, as failure to achieve acceptable compliance with them can affect an organization's accreditation decision.

Intent

The intent describes the purpose and rationale of the standard. This explanation offers the rationale and the context for each standard, providing an explanation of how the standards fit into the overall program. The combined intent statements for all the standards paint a picture of the requirements and goals for IPC.

Measurable Element(s)

Measurable elements of a standard indicate what is reviewed and assigned a score during the survey process. The measurable element(s) for each standard identify the requirements for full compliance with the standard. The measurable elements are intended to bring clarity to the standards and help the organization fully understand the requirements, help educate leaders and staff about the standards, and guide accreditation preparation.

Examples of the standards, intents, and measurable elements are found throughout this book (*see*, for example, Box 2-3 on pages 38–40). The standards are updated approximately every two years based on the ongoing assessment of science, contemporary health care practice, available technology, quality and patient safety practices, and other information.

Components of a Comprehensive IPC Program

The goal of an organization's infection surveillance, prevention, and control program is to identify and reduce the risks of acquiring and transmitting infections among patients, health care workers, contract workers, volunteers, students, and visitors.

IPC programs differ from one organization to another, depending on the organization's geographic location, community, socioeconomic and physical environment, patient volume, populations served, type of clinical activities, and number and education of employees. Effective programs have in common identified leaders, appropriate policies and procedures, staff education, coordination throughout the organization, and systems to identify risks and intervene to minimize or eliminate infections.

The standards are organized into four major sections: Focus, Management, Integration with Quality Improvement and Patient Safety, and Staff Education.

Focus

Standards PCI.1 through PCI.5 describe the organization's responsibilities for determining the focus of the IPC program. PCI.1 emphasizes that the organization designs and implements a coordinated program to reduce the risks of health care–associated (nosocomial) infections in patients and health care workers. For an IPC program to be effective, it must be comprehensive, encompassing both patient care and employee health. Safe, high-quality care for patients and a safe work environment for employees are intertwined because employees and patients who become infected can transmit the infection to other patients or staff. This standard implies a close working relationship between IPC and employee health services.

The IPC program also addresses the infection issues that are epidemiologically important to the organization. This requires assessing risks and key issues that pertain to the particular infections, populations, environment, and other factors that are specific for the organization. In addition, the standard requires that the IPC program is designed to be appropriate to the organization's size, geographic location, services, and patients. A facility that treats primarily trauma patients rather than pediatric or cancer patients or is an ambulatory care center rather than an acute inpatient facility must address the issues most relevant to its patients, services, and setting. Organizations in very rural settings may have challenges that differ from facilities in urban settings. Conditions that should be considered in assessing geographic and environmental influence on infections include the following:

- Natural environmental disruptions—floods, hurricanes, earthquakes, and so forth
- Temperature variations—tropical versus cold
- Vector density—mosquitoes, rodents
- Contaminated water sources or lack of water
- Ecological changes—deforestation, global warming, air pollution, and so forth
- War, migrations, displaced persons
- Urban versus rural—congested housing versus agricultural environments
- Availability, lack of, or disruption of services

The IPC program must involve all patient, staff, and visitor areas of the organization. Because infection can potentially be transmitted by any of the above persons, as well as vendors, volunteers, and students, any of the areas where these persons work should have IPC policies and procedures.

In standard PCI.2, JCI directs the organization to establish the focus of the health care–associated infection prevention and reduction program. Each organization must determine those epidemiologically important infections, infection sites, and associated devices that will provide the focus of efforts to prevent and reduce the incidence of health care– associated infections. Organizations consider, as appropriate, infections that involve the following:

- Urinary tract—such as the invasive procedures and equipment associated with indwelling urinary catheters, urinary drainage systems, and their care
- Surgical wounds (surgical sites)—such as preoperative antimicrobials, operative procedures, care of surgical sites, type of dressing, and associated aseptic procedures
- Respiratory tract—such as the procedures and equipment associated with respiratory therapy, intubation, mechanical ventilatory support, and tracheostomy
- Intravascular invasive devices—such as the insertion and care of central venous catheters and peripheral venous lines

In addition to specific infections, issues such as employee exposures or environmental hazards may be selected as areas that are considered epidemiologically important and should be addressed in planning the focus of the IPC program.

Standard PCI.3 directs the organization to identify procedures and processes associated with the risk of infection and implement strategies to reduce infection risk. Health care organizations assess and care for patients using many simple and complex processes, each associated with a level of infection risk to patients and staff. Thus, it is important for an organization to review those processes and, as appropriate, implement needed policies, procedures, education, and other activities to reduce the risk of infection. Infection risk reduction activities may include, as appropriate to the organization, the following:

- Equipment cleaning and sterilization—in particular, invasive equipment
- Laundry and linen management
- Disposal of infectious waste and body fluids
- Handling and disposal of blood and blood components
- Kitchen sanitation and food preparation and handling
- Operation of the mortuary and postmortem area
- Disposal of sharps and needles
- Separation of patients with communicable diseases from patients and staff who are at greater risk due to immunosuppression or other reasons
- Management of hemorrhagic (bleeding) patients
- Engineering controls, such as positive ventilation systems, biological hoods in laboratories, and thermostats on water heaters
- Cleaning and disinfection of the patient care environment

Because risks can change over time, and sometimes can change quite rapidly, this assessment process should be ongoing. JCI recommends that organizations analyze risks annually or on an "as needed basis" such as when a new program or service is added, a new building is opened, or an organization begins a new service or invasive procedure. In addition, new

---

SIDEBAR 2-1

Addressing IPC Issues Surrounding Visitors

Although health care organizations do not need to track infections in visitors per se, they should be aware of the infections and risks that visitors can bring into an organization or, conversely, be exposed to in an organization. For example, during the severe acute respiratory syndrome (SARS) epidemic in Canada, some organizations stated that they should have moved more quickly to limit visitors, thus reducing the risk of spreading the infection. Visitors to patients with active tuberculosis must use proper barrier precautions, and those visiting high-risk patients (for example, immunocompromised, newborns) should be screened for communicable disease before their visit.

---

patient populations or procedures might introduce new potential infection risks, and an assessment should be conducted whenever new procedures are implemented or populations change.

Any person who enters the health care facility may bring in communicable diseases that can then be transmitted to patients or caregivers. Children may be incubating infections such as varicella or respiratory syncytial virus, and adults could be carrying multidrug-resistant organisms on their wounds or have open pulmonary tuberculosis. Persons visiting patients may also be at risk for acquiring infections from patients or staff. *See* Sidebar 2-1 above for IPC issues related to visitors to a facility.

Standard PCI.4 indicates that gloves, masks, soap, and disinfectants are available and used correctly when required. Hand hygiene materials, barrier techniques, antiseptics, and disinfecting agents are fundamental to IPC. The organization must identify those situations in which masks and gloves are required and ensure that the products are available and accessible. For example, soap, alcohol hand preparations, and disinfectants should be located in those areas where hand hygiene and disinfecting procedures are required. Staff must be educated in proper hand-washing and disinfecting procedures. (For more information on hand hygiene, *see* Box 2-4, pages 42–46, and Appendix 2.)

In standard PCI.5, organizations are instructed to obtain cultures from sites determined to be most associated with significant infection risk (*see* the discussion about standard PCI.3 on page 33 for sites to consider for such surveillance activities). Each organization should identify the sites to be cultured, the rationale for the culture, the frequency of collection, and how the culture results will be interpreted and used before collecting specimens. These cultures may be used to evaluate infection clusters or outbreaks, hemodialysis fluids, or the commissioning of an operating room or new patient area, or to test the effectiveness of cleaning procedures. Individuals responsible for obtaining specimens should be trained in the proper collection and handling of microbiological specimens. Although this is a JCI standard, in the international arena, and particularly in countries with very limited resources, the use of environmental cultures would most likely be limited to an outbreak.

Management

Standards PCI.6 through PCI.10 deal with organizational oversight of the IPC program. PCI.6 indicates that one or more individuals oversee all IPC activities and that the individual(s) is qualified in IPC practices through education, training, experience, or certification. The IPC program has oversight appropriate to the organization's size and the program's scope. One or more individuals, acting on a full-time or part-time basis, provide that oversight. Their qualification depends on the activities they will carry out and may be met through education or training programs, as well as on-the-job experience and certification or licensure. The designation of a particular individual(s) helps in the coordination of the multiple facets of the program. Although decentralization of IPC leadership can be effective, it sometimes leads to gaps in performance and less accountability. The person(s) designated for the oversight role coordinates the dynamics of program management, including how to address changing infection risks and implement intervention strategies, ensures inclusion of all programs and services, and generates policies and procedures to guide compliance with best IPC practices. It is important for this person(s) to be qualified through continuing education and experience to oversee all of the IPC activities.

Standards PCI.7 and PCI.8 discuss program management by designating those persons or groups who coordinate a program. PCI.7 indicates that a designated individual or group monitors and coordinates IPC activities in the organization, and PCI.8 directs that the coordination of IPC activities involves medicine, nursing, and others as appropriate to the organization. IPC activities involve individuals in every department or service who perform nearly every function within a health care organization. One individual or a committee is appointed to coordinate the overall program. Responsibilities include setting criteria to define health care–associated infections, establishing data collection methods, implementing risk reduction strategies, and reporting processes and outcomes. Coordination involves communicating with the entire organization to ensure that the program is continuous and proactive. Medical and nursing staff are represented and engaged in IPC activities, no matter which mechanism is chosen by the organization to coordinate the program. Others who may be included, as determined by the organization's size and services, include the following:

- Epidemiologist, infection control physician, IPC officer, or infection control nurse
- Surveillance or data collection staff
- Statistician
- Central sterilization manager
- Microbiologist

- Pharmacist
- Operating theater supervisor

When the program oversight activities reside with a committee, it is incumbent on the organization to provide each member with education and training, as well as clearly defined roles and responsibilities.

Standards PCI.9 and PCI.10 are concerned with grounding the IPC program in science, regulation, and technology. PCI.9 sets forth that the IPC program is based on current scientific knowledge, accepted practice guidelines, and applicable laws and regulations. Current scientific information is required to understand and implement effective surveillance and control activities; practice guidelines provide information on preventive practices and infections associated with clinical services; and applicable laws and regulations define elements of the basic program and reporting requirements. PCI.10 requires that organization information management systems support the IPC program. Information management systems support the tracking of risks, rates, and trends in health care–associated infections; information management functions support data analysis, interpretation, and presentation of findings; and IPC program data and information are managed with those of the organization's patient safety and quality management and improvement programs.

Organizations must include in their IPC program activities review of evidence-based information from respected organizations, scientific peer-reviewed journals, and other sources. Practice guidelines—such as those for hand hygiene, insertion and care of central lines and other indwelling catheters, and care of the surgical patient before, during and after surgery—should be used to formulate policies and practices. When planning construction or making other environmental alterations, or selecting methods for disinfection or sterilization, local or national rules and regulations and science should be applied to the process.

Integration with Quality Improvement and Patient Safety

Standard PCI.11 and its associated standards are the foundation of JCI's requirement that organizations make certain that IPC measures are given equal weight with other quality improvement measures. PCI.11 requires that the IPC process is integrated with the organization's overall quality improvement and patient safety program. The IPC process is designed to lower the risk of infection for patients, staff, and others. To reach this goal, the organization must proactively monitor and track risks, rates, and trends in health care–associated infections (PCI.11.1).

The organization should also use indicators to monitor infections that are epidemiologically important to the organization (PCI.11.2). If an organization has a large cardiac or neurosurgical surgery service, an extensive neonatal intensive care unit(s), or rehabilitation patients, it should select infection indicators specific for these patient populations. If the organization has a challenging problem with ventilator-associated pneumonia (VAP) in critical care patients, it may choose outcome indicators of infection in populations at risk for VAP for the monitoring or auditing process. Standard PCI.11.3 indicates that risk, rate, and trend information from surveillance, monitoring, or auditing processes are used to design or modify processes to reduce infections to the lowest possible levels. As the information and the associated risks change, the organization must review and modify existing procedures such as those associated with care of the ventilated patient, or the procedures to decrease risk in a surgical patient.

Where possible, an organization should evaluate its IPC data and information by comparing its IPC rates and trends with other similar organizations through comparative databases (PCI.11.4). This process must be carefully designed to ensure that common definitions are used to classify infections as health care associated and that the frequency, intensity, and methods of surveillance are consistent for the comparative organizations. It is important for the IPC program to regularly communicate the results of IPC monitoring to the appropriate staff, physicians, and management (PCI.11.5). The leaders of the organization will use this information to provide guidance to the IPC program staff and to determine priorities and resources allocated to the IPC program. In addition to internal reporting, the organization must disseminate information on infections to the appropriate external public health agencies (PCI.11.6). The recipients will vary among countries. Some countries have a nationwide database on infections; in other countries all information is collected by the ministry of health or other governmental organization.

Staff Education

The last section of the PCI standards requires maintaining a knowledgeable organization staff. PCI.12 states that organizations will provide IPC education to staff, physicians, patients, and, as appropriate or applicable, to family and other caregivers. For an organization to have an effective IPC program, it must educate staff members about the program when they begin work in the organization and regularly thereafter (PCI.12.1). The education program includes professional staff, clinical and nonclinical support staff, and even patients and families, if appropriate. The program may also include tradespeople and other visitors. The education focuses on the policies, procedures, and practices that guide the organization's IPC program. The education also includes the findings and significant trends (PCI.12.2) from the monitoring or auditing activities, new services, or changes in IPC practices.

Other IPC-related standards, intents, and measureable elements are listed in Box 2-3.

Box 2-3

Other Standards Related to Infection Prevention and Control

The standards printed in **bold** typeface are core standards that all organizations must meet to be accredited. These standards are effective as of October 2006, but hospital standards will be updated in 2007.

Facility Management and Safety (FMS)

FMS.5 The organization has a plan for the inventory, handling, storage, and use of hazardous materials and the control and disposal of hazardous materials and waste.
(Applicable to ambulatory care, clinical laboratories [RSM.3.4], care continuum [EMS.6], hospital, and medical transport [BCA.5].)

Intent of FMS.5

The organization identifies and safely controls hazardous materials and waste according to a plan. Such materials and waste include chemicals, chemotherapeutic agents, radioactive materials and waste, hazardous gases and vapors, and other regulated medical and infectious waste. The plan provides processes for

- handling, storage, and use of hazardous materials;
- the inventory of hazardous materials and waste;
- reporting and investigation of spills, exposures, and other incidents;
- proper disposal of hazardous waste;
- proper protective equipment and procedures during use, spill, or exposure;
- documentation, including any permits, licenses, or other regulatory requirements; and
- proper labeling of hazardous materials and waste.

Measurable Elements of FMS.5

1. The organization identifies hazardous materials and waste.
2. Hazardous materials and waste are managed according to a plan.
3. The plan includes safe handling, storage, and use.
4. The plan includes reporting and investigation of spills, exposures, and other incidents.
5. The plan includes the proper disposal of hazardous waste.
6. The plan includes the proper protective equipment and procedures during use, spill, or exposure.
7. The plan identifies documentation requirements including any permits, licenses, or other regulatory requirements.

BOX 2-3—CONTINUED

8. The plan includes labeling hazardous materials and waste.
9. The plan is implemented and followed.

MOI.3 Aggregate data and information support patient care, organization management, and the quality management program.
(Applicable to ambulatory care, hospital, and medical transport [MOI.4].)

The organization collects and analyzes aggregate data to support patient care and organization management. Aggregate data provide a profile of the organization over time and allow the comparison of the organization's performance with other organizations. Thus, aggregate data are an important part of the organization's performance improvement activities. In particular, aggregate data from risk management, utility system management, infection control, and utilization review can help the organization understand its current performance and identify opportunities for improvement. Clinical care providers, researchers, educators, and managers often need information to assist with their responsibilities. Such information may include scientific and management literature, clinical practice guidelines, research findings, and educational methodologies. The Internet, print materials in a library, online search sources, and personal materials are all valuable sources of current information. By participating in external performance databases, an organization can compare its performance to that of other similar organizations locally, nationally, and internationally. Performance comparison is an effective tool for identifying opportunities for improvement and documenting the organization's performance level. Health care networks and those purchasing or paying for health care often ask for such information. External databases vary widely from insurance databases to those maintained by professional societies.

Measurable Elements of MOI.3

1. Aggregate data and information support patient care.
2. Aggregate data and information support organization management.
3. Aggregate data and information support the quality management program.

(continued)

Box 2-3—CONTINUED

Quality Improvement and Patient Safety (QPS)

QPS.3.8 Clinical monitoring includes infection control, surveillance, and reporting.
(Applicable to ambulatory care, continuum of care [QMS.2.7], and hospital.)

An organization's leaders are responsible for making the final selection of the key measures to be included in the organization's monitoring activities. The measures selected relate to the important clinical and managerial areas identified in standards QPS.3.1 through QPS.3.18. For each of these areas, leaders decide

- the process, procedure, or outcome to be measured;
- how measurement will be accomplished; and
- the frequency of measurement.

(Note: Based on the standard, this includes infection control data [QPS 3.8] and data that may be related to infection prevention and control such as surgical procedures [QPS 3.3] and antibiotic use [QPS 3.4].)

Measurable Element of QPS.3.8

1. Clinical monitoring includes the areas identified in the standard.

Source: Joint Commission Resources: *Joint Commission International Accreditation Standards for Hospitals,* Second Edition, 2002. Oakbrook Terrace, IL: Joint Commission on Accreditation of Healthcare Organizations.

Infection Prevention and Control and the International Patient Safety Goals

JCI has presented its first set of International Patient Safety Goals in 2006, including a goal for IPC programs:

> **Goal: Reduce the risk of health care–associated infections.**
> Requirement 7: Comply with current published and generally accepted hand hygiene guidelines.
> **NOTE:** *This should recognize that not all countries have a CDC (Centers for Disease Control and Prevention) or may not recognize the US CDC.*

This International Patient Safety Goal addresses the issue of IPC by suggesting that organizations comply with the WHO's or US CDC's guidelines on hand hygiene, depending on local regulations or preferences. (Although the WHO and US CDC guidelines are suggested as ways to meet this safety goal, an international organization can use another set of guidelines that is "published and generally accepted." This will usually mean guidelines that are evidence based.) According to the US CDC, clean hands are the single most important factor in preventing the spread of dangerous germs and antibiotic resistance in health care settings[1], yet the compliance rate among staff in health care organizations ranges between 25% and 50%.[2,3] There are several reasons that health care workers fail to comply with hand hygiene, including the following:

- Perceived lack of time. According to at least one expert, there is a reverse correlation between how sick patients are on a unit, how busy the unit is, and how frequently caregivers wash their hands.[3]
- Irritation and dryness caused by hand-washing agents
- Belief that gloves eliminate the need for hand hygiene
- Doubt about the value of hand hygiene
- Lack of role models such as colleagues and superiors who engage in frequent hand hygiene[4]

The US CDC (in 2002) and the WHO (in 2005) released new guidelines for hand hygiene in health care settings based on extensive review of the scientific literature and the consensus of world experts. The guidelines advise, among other things, the preferential use of alcohol-based hand rubs for routine hand hygiene, as well as traditional soap and water and sterile gloves when appropriate to protect patients in health care settings. Also included are recommendations for care of the hands, use of artificial nails, and use of gloves, as well as leadership guidelines (*see* Box 2-4, page 42–46).

Box 2-4

World Health Organization (WHO) Guidelines on Hand Hygiene in Health Care

Categories

The WHO has used the same category guidelines for its recommendations as those used by the U.S. Centers for Disease Control/Healthcare Infection Control Practices Advisory Committee. They include the following:

- *Category IA.* Strongly recommended for implementation and strongly supported by well-designed experimental, clinical, or epidemiological studies.
- *Category IB.* Strongly recommended for implementation and supported by some experimental, clinical, or epidemiological studies and a strong theoretical rationale.
- *Category IC.* Required for implementation, as mandated by federal and/or state regulation or standard.
- *Category II.* Suggested for implementation and supported by suggestive clinical or epidemiological studies or a theoretical rationale or a consensus by a panel of experts.

Recommendations

1. Indications for handwashing and hand antisepsis

A. Wash hands with soap and water when visibly dirty or contaminated with proteinaceous material, or visibly soiled with blood or other body fluids, or if exposure to potential spore-forming organisms [such as *Clostridium difficile*] is strongly suspected or proven (IB) or after using the restroom [toilet] (II) [*see* Figure 2-1, page 47].

B. Preferably use an alcohol-based hand rub for routine hand antisepsis in all other clinical situations described in items C.a) to C.f) listed below if hands are not visibly soiled (IA) [*see* Figure 2-2, page 48]. Alternatively, wash hands with soap and water (IB).

C. Perform hand hygiene:
   a) before and after having direct contact with patients (IB);
   b) after removing gloves (IB);
   c) before handling an invasive device (regardless of whether or not gloves are used) for patient care (IB);
   d) after contact with body fluids or excretions, mucous membranes, non-intact skin, or wound dressings (IA);

    e) if moving from a contaminated body site to a clean body site during patient care (IB);

    f) after contact with inanimate objects (including medical equipment) in the immediate vicinity of the patient (IB).

D. Wash hands with either plain or antimicrobial soap and water or rub hands with an alcohol-based formulation before handling medication and preparing food (IB).

E. When alcohol-based hand rub is already used, do not use antimicrobial soap concomitantly (II).

2. Hand hygiene technique

A. Apply a palmful of the product (in a cupped hand) and cover all surfaces of the hands. Rub hands until hands are dry (IB).

B. When washing hands with soap and water, wet hands with water and apply the amount of product necessary to cover all surfaces. Vigorously perform rotational hand rubbing on both palms and interlace fingers to cover all surfaces. Rinse hands with water and dry thoroughly with a single use towel. Use running and clean water whenever possible. Use towel [such as a disposable towel] to turn off faucet (IB).

C. Make sure hands are dry. Use a method that does not recontaminate hands. Make sure towels are not used multiple times or by multiple people (IB). Avoid using hot water, as repeated exposure to hot water may increase the risk of dermatitis (IB).

D. Liquid, bar, leaflet or powdered forms of plain soap are acceptable when washing hands with a non-antimicrobial soap and water. When bar soap is used, small bars of soap in racks that facilitate drainage should be used (II).

3. Recommendations for surgical hand preparation

A. If hands are visibly soiled, wash hands with a plain soap before surgical hand preparation (II). Remove debris from underneath fingernails using a nail cleaner, preferably under running water (II).

B. Sinks should be designed to decrease the risk of splashes (II).

C. Remove rings, watches, and bracelets before beginning surgical hand preparation (II). Artificial nails are prohibited (IB).

D. Surgical hand antisepsis should be performed using either an antimicrobial soap or an alcohol-based hand rub, preferably with sustained activity, before donning sterile gloves (IB).

(continued)

Box 2-4—CONTINUED

E. If quality of water is not assured in the operating theatre, surgical hand antisepsis using an alcohol-based hand rub is recommended before donning sterile gloves when performing surgical procedures (II).

F. When performing surgical hand antisepsis using an antimicrobial soap, scrub hands and forearms for the length of time recommended by the manufacturer, 2 to 5 min. Long scrub times (e.g. 10 min) are not necessary (IB).

G. When using an alcohol-based surgical hand rub product with sustained activity, follow the manufacturer's instructions. Apply the product on dry hands only (IB). Do not combine surgical hand scrub and surgical hand rub with alcohol-based products sequentially (II).

H. When using an alcohol-based product, use sufficient product to keep hands and forearms wet with the hand rub throughout the procedure (IB).

I. After application of the alcohol-based product, allow hands and forearms to dry thoroughly before donning sterile gloves (IB).

4. Selection and handling of hand hygiene agents

A. Provide health-care workers with efficacious hand hygiene products that have low irritancy potential (IB).

B. To maximize acceptance of hand hygiene products by health-care workers, solicit their input regarding the feel, fragrance, and skin tolerance of any products under consideration. In some settings, cost may be a primary factor (IB).

C. When selecting hand hygiene products:
- determine any known interactions between products used to clean hands, skin care products, and the types of gloves used in the institution (II);
- solicit information from manufacturers about risk of contamination (pre-marketing and in-use) (IB);
- ensure that dispensers are accessible at the point of care (IB);
- ensure that dispensers function adequately and reliably, and deliver an appropriate volume of the product (II);
- ensure that the dispenser system for alcohol-based formulations is approved for flammable materials (IC);
- solicit information from manufacturers regarding any effects that hand lotions, creams, or alcohol-based hand rubs may have on the effects of antimicrobial soaps being used in the institution (IB).

D. Do not add soap to a partially empty soap dispenser. If soap dispensers are reused, follow recommended procedures for cleansing (IA).

Box 2-4—CONTINUED

5. Skin care

A. Include information regarding hand care practices designed to reduce the risk of irritant contact dermatitis and other skin damage in health-care workers education programs (IB).

B. Provide alternative hand hygiene products for health-care workers with allergies or adverse reactions to standard products used in the health-care setting (II).

C. When needed to minimize the occurrence of irritant contact dermatitis associated with hand antisepsis or handwashing, provide health-care workers with hand lotions or creams (IA).

6. Use of gloves

A. The use of gloves does not replace the need for hand cleansing by either handrubbing or handwashing (IB).

B. Wear gloves when it can be reasonably anticipated that contact with blood or other potentially infectious materials, mucous membranes, and non-intact skin will occur (IC).

C. Remove gloves after caring for a patient. Do not wear the same pair of gloves for the care of more than one patient (IB).

D. When wearing gloves, change or remove gloves during patient care if moving from a contaminated body site to a clean body site within the same patient or to the environment (II).

E. Avoid reuse of gloves (IB). If gloves are re-used, implement reprocessing methods to ensure glove integrity and microbiological decontamination (II).

7. Other aspects of hand hygiene

A. Do not wear artificial fingernails or extenders when having direct contact with patients (IA).

B. Keep natural nails short (tips less than 0.5 cm long) (II).

8. Health-care worker educational training and motivational programs

A. In hand hygiene promotion programs for health-care workers, focus specifically on factors currently found to significantly influence behavior, and not solely on the type of hand hygiene products. The strategy must be multifaceted and multimodal and include education and senior executive support for implementation (IB).

B. Educate health-care workers about the type of patient-care activities that can result in hand contamination and about the advantages and disadvantages of various methods used to clean hands (II).

(continued)

BOX 2-4—CONTINUED

C. Monitor health-care workers' adherence to recommended hand hygiene practices and provide them with performance feedback (IA).
D. Encourage partnerships between patients, their families, and health-care workers to promote hand hygiene in health care (II).

9. Governmental and institutional responsibilities

9.1 For hospital administrators
A. Provide health-care workers with access to safe continuous water supply at all faucets and access to necessary facilities to perform handwashing (IB).
B. Provide health-care workers with a readily accessible alcohol-based hand rub at the point of patient care (IA).
C. Make improved hand hygiene adherence an institutional priority and provide appropriate leadership, administrative support, and financial resources (IB).
D. Assign health-care professionals with dedicated time and training for the institutional infection control activities, including the implementation of a hand hygiene promotional program (II).
E. Implement a multidisciplinary, multifaceted and multimodal program designed to improve adherence of health-care workers to recommended hand hygiene practices (IB).
F. With regard to hand hygiene, ensure that the water supply within the health-care setting is physically separated from drainage and sewerage, and provide routine system monitoring and management (IB).

9.2 For national governments
A. Make improved hand hygiene adherence a national priority and consider provision of a funded, coordinated, and implemented program for improvement (II).
B. Support strengthening of infection control capacities within health-care settings (II).
C. Promote hand hygiene at the community level to strengthen both self-protection and protection of others (II).

Source: Used with permission from the World Health Organization, *WHO Guidelines on Hand Hygiene in Health Care* (Advanced Draft). Oct. 10, 2005.

Figure 2-1
Handwashing Technique with Soap and Water

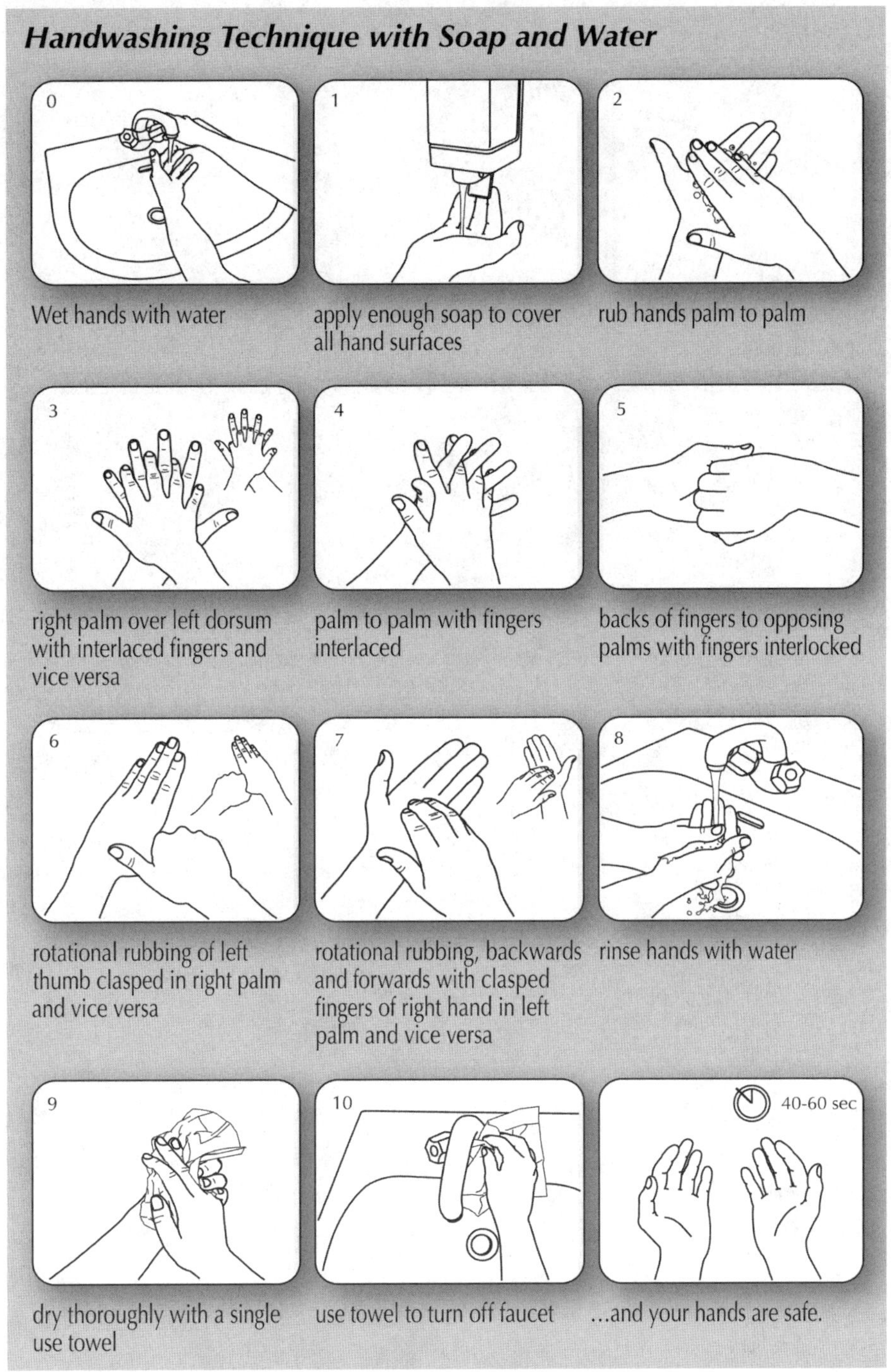

Source: Used with permission from the World Health Organization, *WHO Guidelines on Hand Hygiene in Health Care* (Advanced Draft). Oct. 10, 2005.

Figure 2-2

Hand Hygiene Technique with Alcohol-Based Formulation

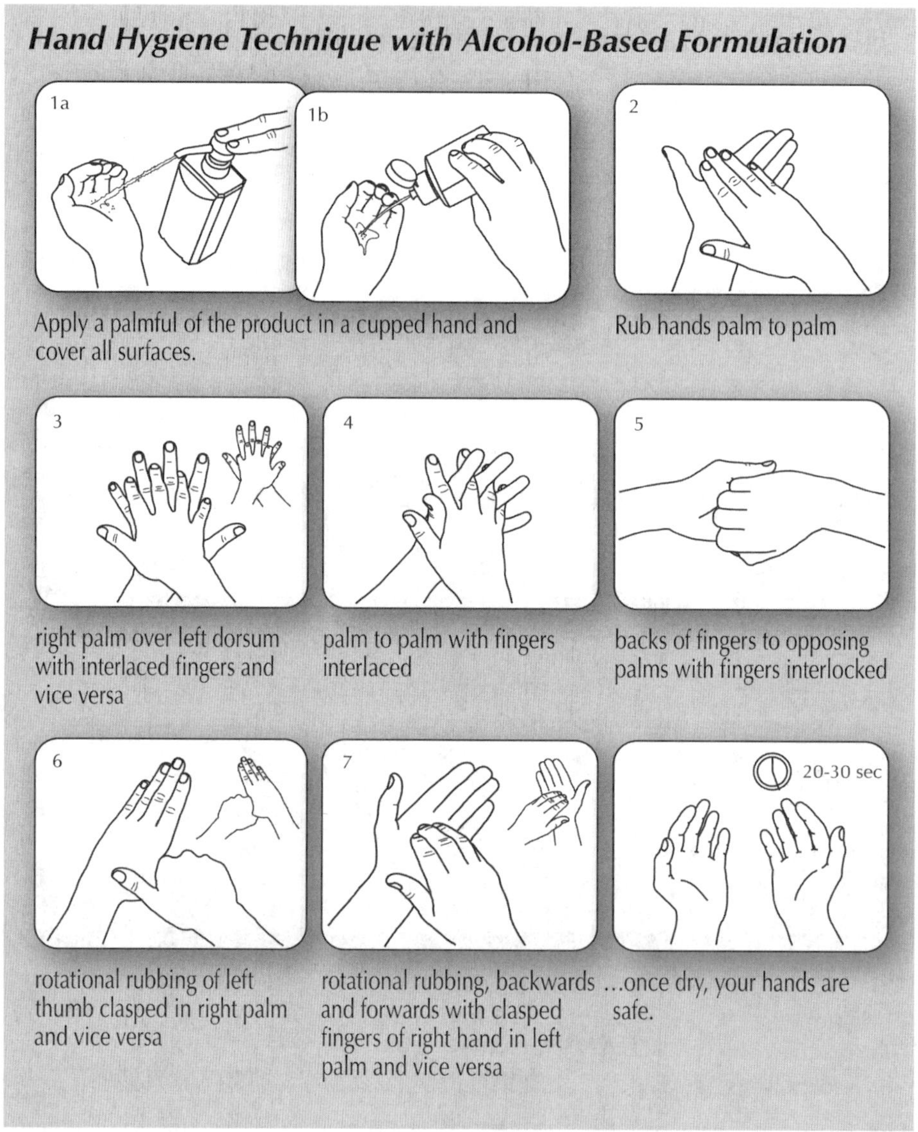

Source: Used with permission from the World Health Organization, *WHO Guidelines on Hand Hygiene in Health Care* (Advanced Draft). Oct. 10, 2005.

For organizations to meet the requirements of the International Patient Safety Goal, all Category I recommendations (including Categories IA, IB, and IC) should be implemented. Category II recommendations should be considered for implementation but are not required for JCI accreditation purposes. However, as stated in Chapter 1, an international organization can use another set of guidelines that is "published and generally accepted." This will usually mean guidelines that are evidence based.

Although the WHO guidelines outline the appropriate use of alcohol-based hand rubs (if hands are not visibly soiled, the use of hand rubs is appropriate and preferred), individuals are not required to use them. However, if an individual chooses not to use them, then he or she should use soap and water instead. Towelettes (for example, paper towels embedded with an antiseptic product such as alcohol) are not a substitute for hand washing, and non–alcohol-based rubs are not recommended.

The guidelines offer appropriate techniques for hand hygiene, including using soap and water for 15 seconds and rubbing the hands together with an alcohol-based hand rub until the hands are dry. The guidelines also cover the appropriate selection of hand hygiene agents, formulas for preparing alcohol-based hand hygiene agents in the organization, and recommendations for appropriate skin care. At the time of this publication, the WHO's guidelines on hand hygiene are being revised and are expected to be made final in 2007. For updates, check the WHO Web site at http://www.who.int.

Some organizations have expressed concern that alcohol-based hand rubs are flammable. Although acknowledging this concern, JCI believes that the typical alcohol gel and foam dispensers in the health care setting are of such limited size and volume that the alcohol gel's contribution to the acceleration of fire development or fire spread is "negligible." In all cases, organizations are advised to consult with and follow the advice of their local fire authorities.

Finally, a note on the International Patient Safety Goals: At the time of this publication, the goals are a part of the JCI hospital survey, but do not affect an organization's accreditation decision. In 2007, the goals will be surveyed and scored.

Institute for Healthcare Improvement's Hand Hygiene Toolkit

The Institute for Healthcare Improvement has collaborated with the US CDC, the Association for Professionals in Infection Control and Epidemiology, and the Society of Healthcare Epidemiology of America to produce *How-to Guide: Improving Hand Hygiene*, a 32-page toolkit that includes tips, forms, and current information for staff members looking to enhance their hand hygiene practices. The toolkit is included in this book as Appendix 2.

References

1. Centers for Disease Control and Prevention: *CDC Releases New Hand-Hygiene Guidelines.* http://www.cdc.gov/handhygiene/pressrelease.htm (accessed Jun. 28, 2006).
2. Lankford M.G., et al.: Influence of role models and hospital design on the hand hygiene of health-care workers. *Emerg Infect Dis* 9, Feb. 2003. http://www.cdc.gov/ncidod/EID/vol9no2/02-0249.htm.
3. Pittet D., Mourouga P., Perneger T.V.: Compliance with handwashing in a teaching hospital. *Ann Intern Med.* 130(2):126–130, Jan. 1999.
4. Boyce J.M., Pittet D.: *Guidelines for Hand Hygiene in Health-Care Settings. Recommendations of the Healthcare Infection Control Practices Advisory Committee and the HICPAC/SHEA/APIC/IDSA Hand Hygiene Task Force.* Centers for Disease Control and Prevention. Oct. 25, 2002. http://www.cdc.gov/mmwr/preview/mmwrhtml/rr5116a1.htm.

Further Readings

Boyce J.M., et al.: Lack of association between the increased incidence of *clostridium difficile*-associated disease and the increasing use of alcohol-based hand rubs, *Infect Control Hosp Epidemiol* 27:479–483, May 2006.

Donahue K.T., vanOstenberg P.: Joint Commission International accreditation: Relationship to four models of evaluation *Intl J Qual Health Care,* 12(3):243–246, 2000.

Heidemann, E.G.: Moving to global standards for accreditation processes: The ExPeRT Project in a larger context. *Int J Qual Health Care* 12(3):227–230, 2000.

Huber M.A., Holton R.H., Terezhalmy G.T.: Cost analysis of hand hygiene using antimicrobial soap and water versus an alcohol-based hand rub. *J Contemp Dent Pract* 7:37–45, May 2006.

Kusachi S., et al.: Creating a manual for proper hand hygiene and its clinical effects. *Surg Today* 36(5):410–415, 2006.

Oh H.S., et al.: National survey of the status of infection surveillance and control programs in acute care hospitals with more than 300 beds in the Republic of Korea. *Am J Infect Control* 34:223–233, May 2006.

Patarakul K., et al.: Cross-sectional survey of hand-hygiene compliance and attitudes of health care workers and visitors in the intensive care units at King Chulalongkorn Memorial Hospital. *J Med Assoc Thai* 88 (suppl. 4):S287–S293, Sep. 2005.

Shimokura G., et al.: Factors associated with personal protection equipment use and hand hygiene among hemodialysis staff. *Am J Infect Control* 34:100–107, Apr. 2006.

vanOstenberg P.: Quality measurement across borders: needs and options. *World Hosp Health Serv* 42(1):19–22, 2006.

Resources

The following readings were gathered for use in *Information Resources in Infection Control,* Fourth Edition (Editor: Nizam Damani M.D., MBBS, MSc, FRCPI, FRCPath), due in 2006 from the International Federation of Infection Control (IFIC). The full document will be available online at IFIC's Web site: http://www.theific.org/publications.asp. NOTE: Some of these resources may appear at the end of more than one chapter, due to their applicability to more than one aspect of infection prevention and control.

Arias, K., Soule, B. (eds.): *The APIC/JCAHO Infection Control Workbook.* Washington, D.C., and Oakbrook Terrace, IL: Association for Professionals in Infection Control and Epidemiology, Inc., and Joint Commission on Accreditation of Healthcare Organizations, 2006.

Department of Health (UK): *Saving Lives: A Delivery Programme to Reduce Healthcare Associated Infections Including MRSA.* London: Department of Health, 2005. http://www.dh.gov.uk/PublicationsAndStatistics/ Publications/PublicationsLibrary/fs/en.

————: *Audit Tools for Monitoring Infection Control Standards.* London: Department of Health, 2004. http://www.dh.gov.uk/PublicationsAndStatistics/ Publications/PublicationsLibrary/fs/en.

Health Canada: Infection control guidelines: Hand washing, cleaning, disinfection and sterilization in health care. *Can Commun Dis Rep* 24S8 (suppl.), Dec. 1998.

Hospital Infection Society, Infection Control Nurses Association, Department of Health (UK): *Working Group Report. Key Indicators in Infection Control.* 2004. http://www.his.org.uk/_db/_documents/keyindicators2002- 2003jan2004.pdf.

Infection Control Nurses Association (ICNA): Hand Decontamination Guidelines. Bathgate, UK: ICNA, 2002.

————: *Competencies Self-Assessment Tool.* 2001. http://www.icna.co.uk (user name and password required).

Infection Control Nurses Association and Department of Health (UK): *Audit Tools for Monitoring Infection Control Guidelines Within Community.* (Book and CD ROM.) Bathgate, UK: Fitwise, 2005.

————: *Audit Tools for Monitoring Infection Control Standards 2004* (Book and CD ROM.) Bathgate, UK: Fitwise, 2004.

Joint Commission Resources: *Meeting JCAHO's Infection Control Requirements: A Priority Focus Area.* Oakbrook Terrace, IL: Joint Commission on Accreditation of Healthcare Organizations, 2004.

Labadie J.C., et al.: Recommendation for surgical hand disinfection— Requirements, implementation and need for research: A proposal by representatives of the SFHH, DGHM and DGKH for a European discussion. *J Hosp Infect* 51:312–315, Mar. 2002.

Malik R.E., Cooper R.A., Griffith C.J.: Use of audit tools to evaluate the efficacy of cleaning systems in hospitals. *Am J Infect Control* 31(3):181–187, 2003.

Society for Healthcare Epidemiology of America: An approach to the evaluation of quality indicators of the outcome of care in hospitalized patients, with a focus on nosocomial infection indicators. *Infect Control Hosp Epidemio* 16(5):308–316, 1995. http://www.shea-online.org/publications/shea_position_papers.cfm.

Strategy for the Control of Antimicrobial Resistance in Ireland (SARI) Infection Control Subcommittee: *Guidelines for Hand Hygiene in Irish Health Care Settings.* 2004. http://www.ndsc.ie/A-Z/Gastroenteric/ Handwashing/Publications/File,1047,en.pdf.

Surveying Infection Prevention and Control

The Role of Infection Prevention and Control in the Accreditation Survey Process

The surveillance, prevention, and control of infections affects every part of an organization and every aspect of patient care and employee safety. Lack of attention in this area can lead to decreased patient safety, adverse events, tremendous organizational expense, and ultimately an unsafe organization. Because it has a significant impact on an organization's provision of safe and high-quality care, it is not surprising that infection prevention and control (IPC) is evaluated in multiple ways during the accreditation process. This chapter offers a brief look at the Joint Commission International (JCI) accreditation process specifically for IPC and offers examples for compliance readiness. The IPC portion of the JCI survey consists of two main activities: the infection control interview and a review of IPC policies and practices throughout the organization through interaction with staff, departments, and services and, beginning in 2007, through the tracer methodology.

The Infection Control Interview

The IPC portion of the survey process may take only a limited portion of the time of a complete JCI on-site survey (*see* Figure 3-1 on page 54), but the infection control interview is an important part of the process. The interview is JCI's window into the organization's IPC practices, systems and overall competency. The purpose of the infection control interview is to assess the processes used to do the following:

- Develop the IPC program
- Reduce risk and incidence of health care–associated infections

FIGURE 3-1

Joint Commission International Sample Survey Agenda
(4 Days, 3 Surveyors)

DAY ONE

	Physician	Nurse	Administrator
07:45 – 08:15	Opening Conference		
08:15 – 08:45	Hospital's Overview of Organization Services		
08:45 – 10:45	Document Review		
10:45 – 12:00	Leadership Interview		
12:00 – 13:00	Lunch		
13:00 – 15:00	Patient Unit Visit	Patient Unit Visit	Facility Tour
15:00 – 17:00	Anesthetizing Locations Visits	Operating Room, Post-anesthesia Recovery Room	

DAY TWO

	Physician	Nurse	Administrator
08:00 – 08:30	Debriefing		
08:30 – 10:30	Emergency Services Interview	Patient Unit Visit	Facility Tour
10:30 – 12:30	Patient Unit Visit Intensive Care Unit	Patient Unit Visit	Review of Facility Management and Safety Documents
12:30 – 13:30	Lunch with Medical Staff	Lunch with Nursing Leadership	Lunch with CEO
13:30 – 15:00	Imaging Services Visits	Infection Control Interview	Pharmacy Visit
15:00 – 17:00	Staff Qualifications and Education Interview for Medical Staff	Staff Qualifications and Education Interview for Nursing Personnel	Staff Qualifications and Education Interview for other Hospital Personnel

DAY THREE

	Physician	Nurse	Administrator
08:00 – 08:30		Debriefing	
08:30 – 10:30	Patient Unit Visit or Optional Document Review	Patient Unit Visit or Optional Document Review	Patient Unit Visit or Optional Document Review
10:30 – 12:30	Patient Records Interview		Management of Information Interview
12:30 – 13:30	Lunch		
13:30 – 15:00	Quality Improvement and Patient Safety Interview		
15:00 – 17:00	Pathology and Clinical Laboratory Visit	Patient Unit Visit	Rehabilitation Services Visit

DAY FOUR

	Physician	Nurse	Administrator
08:00 – 08:30	Debriefing		
08:30 – 10:00	Patient Unit Visit	Patient Unit Visit	Patient Unit Visit
10:00 – 12:00	Patient Care Interview		
12:00 – 13:00	Working Lunch		
13:00 – 15:00	Integrate Findings		
15:00 – 16:30	Leadership Exit Interview		

- Ensure that IPC personnel are qualified
- Improve performance in IPC, as appropriate to the organization's priorities

The interview is normally held in a small meeting room at the discretion of the hospital leadership. Participants should include the following:

- The individual(s) responsible for the IPC program (for example, the infection control physician and/or infection control nurse)
- Staff involved in implementing the infection prevention and control program (for example, nurses, support staff, environmental services)
- Other staff you may choose (for example, facilities staff, organizational leaders)
- Nurse surveyor

The JCI surveyor(s) facilitating the interview explains its purpose. Participants are asked to explain the components of the organization's IPC program, such as the surveillance and outbreak investigation procedures, education for staff, integration of IPC with quality improvement and patient safety. He or she may ask the team to provide examples of how care is managed for a patient with an infection or at risk of acquiring an infection, reviewing care processes from the time the patient enters the organization until the time he or she exits. The surveyor(s) may also ask about systems issues (for example, information management, occupational health, environmental procedures) that support the IPC program.

The surveyor(s) will also ask about specific issues he or she has identified during the visits to patient care units or settings or during earlier interviews. The surveyor(s) may also ask the IPC team questions that he or she did not have time to ask during the visits to patient care units or settings.

The IPC program and team can prepare for the interview with three simple but significant steps:

1. Know the standards.
2. Make available the proper documents.
3. Practice discussing the program elements.

Standards necessary to demonstrate IPC compliance include the following:

- Standards from the "Prevention and Control of Infections" (PCI) chapter
- Select standards from the following:
  - "Facility Management and Safety" (FMS) chapter (for example, FMS.5)
  - "Management of Information" (MOI) chapter (for example, MOI.1.9 and MOI.3)
  - "Quality Improvement and Patient Safety" (QPS) chapter (for example, QPS.3.8)

See Chapter 2, especially Box 2-3 on pages 38–40, for more information on JCI infection prevention and control standards.

Documents you should have on hand include the following:
- Minutes of IPC committee meetings and other key meetings such as patient safety or performance improvement work involving IPC or departmental or service meetings to discuss IPC issues
- Assessment process and report used to determine the focus and risks of the IPC program
- The IPC plan for the year being surveyed
- Outcome surveillance reports that include data, trends, comparisons, analyses
- Quality improvement reports showing IPC involvement in quality improvement projects
- Key policies and procedures as requested
- Records of education provided to staff
- Records of biological testing

These documents can also be included in the document review session.

To practice for the interview, have another of your organization's staff members ask the IPC staff members and others who will be present at the interview questions about the IPC program. Prepare to discuss how quality management has been able to use IPC surveillance data to lower the risk of health care–acquired infections in the organization and how IPC and environmental health personnel work together to provide a safe environment for patients and follow-up for employee exposures. Be ready to talk about the relationship between facilities management and IPC in relation to construction, renovation, and alterations of the facility and how IPC interacts with key support services such as nutrition and dietary, housekeeping, central sterile supply, and others. For additional preparation, list all of the measures of success and evaluate compliance with each one, indicating an action plan to achieve compliance where gaps exist.

Tracer Methodology

Tracer methodology is an evaluation method that traces the care of a patient while in a health care organization or traces processes that deliver that care. It is currently a part of the JCI on-site survey, but results of tracers will not affect accreditation decisions until 2007. Until then, tracers are an excellent tool for assessing and improving the functions of the IPC program throughout the organization and can be used by IPC programs on a regular basis for monitoring the effectiveness of the program. The purpose of the tracers during the survey will be to assess the quality and safety of the care, treatment, and services related to IPC that are provided by an organization and, thus, its compliance with JCI standards.

The most thorough examination of tracer methodology is found in the Joint Commission Resources 2004 book *Tracer Methodology: Tips and*

Strategies for Continuous Systems Improvement. Because that book is mostly an examination of United States–based procedures and scenarios, much of the following information drawn from that source has been adapted for use in global health care settings.

Individual Tracers

The individual tracer is an evaluation method designed to trace the care experiences of a patient while receiving services from a health care organization. In an individual tracer, a surveyor or surveyor team follows a specific patient through an organization's processes. The surveyor or surveyor team examines the individual components of many systems, such as infection prevention and control, medication administration, care planning, support services, such as laboratory and radiology, and use of data for patient care. In other words, a surveyor or team looks at how each department/unit/program and service provides treatments, services, and patient care as well as how apartments/units/programs and services work together to provide the highest quality of care for the patient.

Systems and measure to prevent infection are part of individual tracers. For example, surveyors may trace a patient having a total hip replacement. In addition to the patient evaluation, teaching, and care planning, surveyors will look at how the surgical process is managed, how drugs are delivered, how intravenous lines are placed and maintained, and how the surgical site is monitored and dressings changed if appropriate. Each of these processes integrates IPC as part of the care that is provided to the patient.

Individual tracers are the primary focus of the on-site survey process. They are used to examine all aspects of care experienced by the patient. Such tracers have many dimensions and might or might not have been selected for a reason related to IPC. However, all individual tracers address IPC issues as relevant and actively engage the front-line staff and physicians in discussion about their roles in IPC and the methods used to prevent or manage infections in patients. Sidebars 3-1 and 3-2 (beginning on page 59) provide examples of individual IPC tracers. Following is a brief discussion of how IPC can influence the selection of individual tracers in a variety of settings, as well as some sample individual tracers. (Note: Although these examples are informative and could provide a means for organizations to prepare for what to expect during an on-site tracer during a survey, it is important to keep in mind that these examples are not necessarily the way that surveyors will conduct a tracer. Each tracer follows a path that is specific and appropriate to the identified areas of focus relevant to your organization.)

- In the hospital setting, a patient might be selected who has or is at risk for a health care–associated infection or a community infection. For example, surveyors may select a patient from the community with active tuberculosis or meningococcal infection to evaluate admission and management processes or a patient in the medical intensive care unit and discuss with staff members how they work to prevent infections in patients on ventilators. Or surveyors may select a surgical patient on the general surgery unit who has a wound infection, and who is on isolation, and ask staff to describe the procedures to prevent spread of the infection. Or surveyors might choose a patient with post–cesarean section with endometritis who is being given antimicrobial agents and will be monitored for recovery before going home.

- Ambulatory care tracers can focus on high-volume or high-risk diagnoses such as certain types of postoperative infections. Patients receiving infusion therapy, blood component administration, chemotherapy, dialysis, indwelling devices, pain management pumps, HIV testing, or vaccine use can all be traced. Clinics that serve patients with tuberculosis or see patients with possible cholera may be reviewed. Surveyors may ask staff members how they recognize symptoms and syndromes (for example, rash, fevers, gastrointestinal symptoms, and so forth), how the patient—and sometimes the family—are managed in the ambulatory setting, and how they report them for follow-up. Hand hygiene and patient education are important. Any tracer, even if not primarily chosen for IPC, may cover these and other IPC components.

System Tracers

System tracers are not a component of JCI's accreditation process and are not expected to be in the near future, but the methodology can be valuable to a health care organization for assessing the IPC program (or any other program). As in an individual tracer, a surveyor performing a system tracer follows a specific patient through his or her course of care. But instead of reviewing all components of the health care delivery system in relation to that patient's care (as is done during an individual tracer), the surveyor evaluates all aspects of a particular system such as IPC. This type of tracer is an in-depth look at a system as it affects the delivery of health care.

The surveyors evaluate and explore the organization's strengths and areas of concern, the integration of related processes, and the coordination and communication among disciplines and departments in those processes related to the system being followed.

IPC, along with medication management and data use, are system issues that will be addressed during the survey process. The topic of IPC can surface in any one of these system tracers. Following is a discussion of three system tracers and how IPC relates to them.

SIDEBAR 3-1

Individual Tracer Example:
Surgical Site Infection in a Hospital Setting

This tracer example might start at any place in the hospital. It starts small and expands as the care systems that have meaning to the patient begin to unfold. During the tracer, surveyors might want to speak with the infection prevention and control (IPC) leaders if infection risk and vulnerabilities have been found or if there is surveillance data related to tracer findings. The following tracer is one example, and although it may not be applicable to your health care setting or identified areas of focus during the survey, it provides a model that conveys the general tracer process.

The Patient

The patient is a 67-year-old male who has had a coronary artery bypass and has developed a surgical site infection five days postsurgery. The surveyors begin the tracer.

Preoperative Care Area

This type of tracer could start in a preoperative area, where the surveyors discuss the preoperative workup with the physicians and nurses. Such elements as ensuring diabetic control, assessing for remote infection such as urinary tract infection, and ensuring preoperative hygiene could be discussed. The surveyors may ask how timely prophylactic preoperative antibiotic dosing is ensured: What is the policy? What is the compliance?

The Patient's Room

The tracer could start or could continue in the patient's room where the surveyors will observe care and treatment on the clinical unit and interview the patient and/or family. The surveyors might perform the following tasks:

- Observe the environment of care and talk to the housekeeper, maintenance, laundry, or dietary personnel on the patient's care unit.
- Review the patient's medical record with the front-line caregiver present. The interdisciplinary care plan and the care plan process could be reviewed as well.
- Ask about dressing change and wound care protocols, checking to see if the procedure matches the policy and assessing the competency of the caregiver
- Probe how the medical staff utilizes the infectious disease physician for diagnosis and treatment and the pharmacy for antibiotic appropriateness

Laboratory

In the laboratory, discussion with staff could include antibiogram use and timely collection, processing, and reporting of culture specimens. Sensitivity to trends and syndromes, as well as the blood culture contamination rate, may be discussed.

(continued)

SIDEBAR 3-1—CONTINUED

Surgical Suite

In the surgical suite, surveyors coordinate their activities so that there will be limited intrusions during the daily work. The following areas might be covered:

- Surgical staff could be asked to confirm that prophylactic antibiotic dosing is performed per policy.
- Surveyors may observe preoperative hand hygiene and confirm that preoperative skin prep protocols are observed.
- Staff may be asked how trends in surgical site infections are identified and actually used. Surgical staff members may also be asked to discuss their interactions with the IPC practitioner and committee, performance improvement personnel, and patient safety personnel.
- Traffic control, air flow, air quality, and other environmental considerations such as the use of quality check lists could be explored.
- Flash autoclave logs may be reviewed, as well as the adequacy of instrument inventory to avoid unnecessary flash autoclave use and the policy for the reuse of disposables.

The Sterile Processing Area

In this department autoclave logs may be examined, as well as the separation of dirty equipment from clean equipment and adherence to aseptic techniques. Inventory, storage, air control, traffic flow or patterns/control, and relative humidity are also important topics. Usually, only one surveyor will visit to avoid multiple intrusions.

Other Care Sites

Other sites associated with the hospital may be involved in this tracer. There may be a long term care unit or facility associated with the hospital ambulatory care clinics, home care components, or a behavioral health care unit that requires surgical site follow-up. In these care areas, the surveyor will observe care and treatment as it might relate to the selected tracer patient. The surveyors could also interview rehabilitation and recreation staff regarding their knowledge of IPC precautions and of reporting infections. Hand hygiene compliance in these other areas, as well as wound care, hygiene, sanitation, patient education, and so forth, can be explored.

SIDEBAR 3-2

More Individual Tracer Examples

Catheter-Related Bloodstream Infection

This tracer can be selected for any program/care location because central lines are used outside of critical care areas as well as in the intensive care unit. If possible, the patient will be interviewed to ascertain what safety teaching took place. Actual line and site care and protocols may be explored. The medical record will be reviewed with the caregiver, as will the care plan. Consistent adherence to facility policies and staff competency could be explored. Timely notice of signs and symptoms of local and systemic infection is an issue, as is timely and competent blood culture collection. Timely, appropriate, antimicrobial dosing and adherence to World Health Organization or U.S. Centers for Disease Control and Prevention guidelines for the placement of central lines could be discussed. Surveyors may review physician response when called with bloodstream infection symptoms.

Urinary Catheter Infection

Indwelling urinary catheters are used primarily in acute and long term care health care settings and are a logical selection for a tracer. The surveyors will view the care and treatment and the condition of the device—Is it on the floor? Is there a leak (normally, an odor will be a sign of a leak)? Is it secured properly below the level of the bladder? to name a few. The patient/family could be interviewed regarding the education they were given about the care of the urinary catheter, the IPC implications, and patient safety. Following are some additional issues the surveyors may address:

- Is the drainage system open or closed?
- If leg bags and night bags are used at intervals, are the protocols for disinfecting/cleaning bags consistent with accepted practices?
- Do nurses and other front-line caregivers know the signs and symptoms of urinary tract infection in the elderly and in the noncommunicative?
- What protocols are in place to assess urinary output?
- Is intermittent catheterization used and under what circumstances? What is the policy?
- What are the protocols for urine culture and sensitivity testing, reporting results to the physician, and treatment response time?
- How does the staff obtain urine specimens and empty urine foley bags?
- What is the policy for the removal of an indwelling urinary catheter?

Cesarean Section

Many of the questions used for a tracer for a surgical patient can be used for a woman undergoing a cesarean section. In addition, surveyors may ask the following:

- How is information about prenatal care provided to the staff?

(continued)

SIDEBAR 3-2—CONTINUED

- What is the process for checking the patient for gestational diabetes or high blood pressure associated with pregnancy?
- How is the woman evaluated for infections that may affect the infant such as HIV, hepatitis, group B streptococcus?
- How and when are antibiotics administered for the C-section procedure?
- How is the patient evaluated for possible post–C-section complications?

Pneumococcal Vaccine for At-Risk Patients

This vaccine is of interest in ambulatory care, primary health care settings, long term care, home care, behavioral health care, adult day care, pediatrics, and so forth. It would probably be selected as a secondary issue in a patient tracer. The organization's policy for identifying the need for the vaccine and administering it will be reviewed and the medical record will be checked for a record of vaccine administration. Performance improvement data for the success of the program could be reviewed.

IPC Tracer

The IPC tracer critically observes and analyzes the organization's IPC program. Potential risk points in the program are identified, and the surveyors might engage the staff in discussion of areas for improvement and actions that can be taken.

The surveyors may explore several areas such as surveillance and infection identification, prevention and control strategies, reporting internally and externally, and education. A hypothetical adverse event could be reviewed. Also, there might be data in the facility that reflect the monetary cost as well as the morbidity and mortality of health care–associated infections, and the surveyors may ask to see these data.

Regardless of the type of tracer, certain key people should be involved. These individuals should be selected for their ability to address issues related to the IPC program in all major departments or areas within the organization. Following is a list of some of the people who may be involved:

- Clinical staff directly involved in the provision of care, treatment, and services, including nurses, physicians, therapists, and pharmacists, as applicable
- Support staff (for example, nutrition and dietetics, radiology)
- Staff responsible for the environment (for example, housekeeping, maintenance)
- IPC staff and organization leadership

This system tracer may begin in an area where care is delivered. The surveyors choose the starting location based on presurvey information and materials reviewed during the planning session (surveillance data, minutes, and reports).

In complex organizations where more than one JCI manual applies, a single IC tracer can review the services throughout the organization. The boundaries of the tracer can expand as needed to encompass ambulatory care, the clinical laboratory, medical transport, and other areas.

The surveyors attempt to assess the staff's knowledge and expectations regarding the IPC program. Surveyors will evaluate staff knowledge of the formal IPC plan and goals. Another outcome is assessing whether or not IPC safety permeates all parts of the organization.

Questions posed to the staff could take the form of scenarios to assess knowledge of and compliance with protocols for the following:

- Hand hygiene and compliance with hand hygiene on their unit or department
- Reporting signs and symptoms of infection, including infection in the cognitively impaired
- Routine precautions and isolation (airborne, droplet, and contact) to prevent spread of disease
- Authority to isolate
- Dressing changes and IV line and site care
- Knowledge and use of trended IPC data, including cross-infection
- Knowledge of resistant organisms and trends
- Knowledge of employee health protocols
- Education of staff for IPC
- Patient and family education regarding preventing infections

The surveyors move from setting to setting, as appropriate, to trace IPC processes across the organization. The clinical staff, physicians who provide direct care, and support staff are interviewed.

Surveyors may visit major specialty areas with populations who are at risk for health care–associated infections, or areas that support the IPC program could be visited. Some of these areas could include the following:

- Preoperative areas (preoperative prophylactic antibiotic dosing, control of diabetes, personal hygiene, changing or removing bladder catheters)
- Surgical department (operating theater) (consistent scrub and prep protocols, air flow and humidity, traffic, antibiotic prophylaxis redosing, trended data use for postoperative infections, infectious disease consults, management of medical equipment general asepsis, and so forth)
- Outpatient surgery/procedural clinics—endoscopy, cardiac catheter, procedural radiology, and so forth (preparation protocols, equipment cleaning, disinfection, sterilization, storage, cleaning the environment and so forth)
- Inpatient psychiatry units and clinics (vaccine, HIV testing, hygiene, sanitation, multipurpose rooms and isolation)

- Rehabilitation departments (with issues such as sanitation, reporting possible infections, dressing or change procedures)
- Pharmacy (antibiogram use in pharmacy and therapeutics committee, interventional pharmacology)
- Laboratory (use of lab data trending, blood culture protocols, blood culture contamination rate, use of antibiograms, strategies for preventing the emergence of resistant strains, timely reporting, syndromes/public health concerns, and so forth)
- Sterile processing (sterilization logs, flash sterilization, turnaround time for specialty packs and adequacy of instruments, storage system, delineated clean and dirty areas, air flow and humidity, traffic patterns, dress code)
- Dietary (general food sanitation protocols, storage, preparation, transport)
- Laundry (general laundry sanitary procedures, temperatures of equipment)
- Employee health clinic (preventive protocols, exposure protocols, and so forth)

The IC system tracer also includes a short group meeting that includes those persons responsible for the program (the IPC practitioners and infectious disease physicians). Depending on your organization, this group might also include risk management, performance or quality improvement, patient safety officers, staff development, and employee health. The discussion may head in any direction. Surveyors will not follow a predetermined set of questions or issues (depending on your organization), but what follows are some of the questions that might be discussed. (Note: these are similar to the questions that would be asked in the infection control interview.)

- How does the IPC program integrate into the facility's culture of safety and quality of care? Questions come from previous visits and interviews with staff.
- How ready is the organization for emerging pathogens such as severe acute respiratory syndrome (SARS) or pandemic avian influenza? For example, is there a cogent plan to assess equipment and supplies and staff capabilities to support containment efforts?
- What is the information technology support for the IPC program? For example, is there a capacity to improve surveillance of health care–associated infections and syndromes of public health interest?
- What is the role of leadership in the program and the long-term commitment for resources? Surveyors will attempt to assess the use of IPC results as reported to the safety committee, chief

executive, board of directors, performance or quality, risk management, peer review, and credentialing group.

- What is the staffing mix of caregivers and support staff, as well as what staff supports the IPC program? What training has been delivered and what is the competency of the IPC program leaders and their authority to act in the face of a perceived threat?
- What efforts are the program and medical staff making to limit the emergence of microbial resistance?
- What is the organization's understanding of the IPC-related International Patient Safety Goal?
- Does the written IPC plan describe the IPC program and the way the organization tracks goals and objectives? Does the plan include the focus and risk assessment of the program? Are trends identified, and are there strategies and actions to control risks?
- What are some of the coming threats, hazard vulnerabilities, and other issues that the organization anticipates?
- How are critical data collated and used? Examples include ventilator-associated pneumonia expressed per 1,000-ventilator days, central line–associated blood stream infections per 1,000-device days, surgical site infections compared internally and externally where feasible, response to syndrome identification and community outbreaks, mortality related to infections, laboratory data related to the program, and so forth.
- How does the organization compare its IPC data and rates to internal and external benchmarks?
- What is IPC's relationship with employee health, dietary, housekeeping, maintenance, laundry, new construction or renovation, and so forth?
- How do surveillance methods produce the types of data needed to guide decision making for IPC issues?
- What methods are used to monitor compliance with the hand hygiene guidelines of the World Health Organization (WHO) (or U.S. Centers for Disease Control and Prevention)?

Data Use Tracer

Risk points in the IPC program can be identified in the data use systems tracer. Items for discussion when IPC is part of the data use system tracer can include the following:

- How are IPC data provided to leaders, staff, physicians, other safety committees, external entities, and so forth?
- How does the information technology function support IPC data collection and analysis?
- How are IPC data integrated with other quality and patient safety data?

Participants in the data use tracer can include (but are not limited to) representatives from the following areas:

- Leadership
- Performance improvement
- Employee health and safety
- Facility or environment of care director
- IPC program leaders
- Information management
- Laboratory
- Nurses
- Pharmacy
- Physicians
- Staff development

Note: The aforementioned list may vary depending on which system tracers are conducted and the size and complexity of the organization.

Medication Management Tracer

The overall goal of the medication management tracer is to facilitate critical thinking about medication system risk points; therefore, the medication management tracer can contain IPC elements, including the following:

- How are physicians trained regarding antibiotic use and the trends of use as viewed by the pharmacy and therapeutics committee or leadership, as well as peer review activities?
- What are the roles of the pharmacy and laboratory in the review of antibiotic use? How are the results of reviews transmitted to the IPC program?
- Are there antibiotic stewardship and facility antibiotic use guidelines, including broad-spectrum antibiotic use guidelines? This could include formulary restrictions or laboratory sensitivity reports for certain antibiotics.
- Are there policies and procedures for managing potentially harmful antibiotic/food/drug interactions prevention?
- How does the organization determine and monitor preoperative antibiotic prophylaxis protocols? How are the results transmitted to the IPC program?
- What is the role of the laboratory in antibiotic use (timely collection, processing, and reporting of urinalysis, cultures [particularly blood cultures], and so forth)?

The tracer methodology is process driven. It is customized for each system or patient traced. The tracers are followed across all services and programs with multilevel participation. The tracer methodology provides a forum for discussion, education, identification of vulnerabilities in systems, and reinforcement of system strengths.

Surveying the International Patient Safety Goal

Although the International Patient Safety Goal related to IPC (*see* Chapter 2) does not fall within the body of the PCI standards, it is currently being surveyed by JCI and will be a survey requirement starting in 2007. It is thus worth considering when preparing for an on-site survey. The emphasis of this evaluation is consistent performance of the requirement, not on documentation or intent. Organizations do not need to create any extra documentation for JCI that they would not already be creating while implementing this goal.

There are a number of ways organizations can assess compliance with the goal. The following list provides examples of particular ways surveyors can assess the goal:

- Determine whether staff are informed about the WHO's hand hygiene guidelines (for example, policy, education, notices, signs).
- Assess the level of staff understanding of the guidelines through observation or interviews.
- Observe implementation of the guidelines.

Conclusion

JCI's accreditation process calls on health care organizations to shift their mindset from viewing accreditation as a single event in time that provides a somewhat narrow and time-sensitive understanding of how well an organization's systems work together to seeing it more as a continuing dynamic and unfolding process that provides insight into the organization's daily operations. JCI addresses IPC at many points during the survey process to determine how organizations incorporate IPC practices into their daily operations and thus help enhance patient and staff safety.

Further Readings

Jepsen O.B.: Towards European Union standards in hospital infection control. *J Hosp Infect* 30 (suppl.):64–68, Jun. 1995.

Joint Commission International Center for Patient Safety: *International Patient Safety Goals Announced.* http://www.jcipatientsafety.org/show.asp?durki=11753&site=164&return=9335.

Joint Commission Resources: *Tracer Methodology: Tips and Strategies for Continuous Systems Improvement.* Oakbrook Terrace, IL: Joint Commission on Accreditation of Healthcare Organizations, 2004.

———: Tying in the environment of care. *Environment of Care News* 7:11, Sep. 2004.

———: Questions and answers about tracer methodology. *Joint Commission: The Source* 2:11, Jul. 2004.

Sax H., Ruef C., Widmer A.F.: Quality standards for hospital hygiene in intermediate and large hospitals in Switzerland: A recommended concept *Schweiz Med Wochenschr* 129:276–284, Feb. 20, 1999.

Resources

The following readings were gathered for use in *Information Resources in Infection Control,* Fourth Edition (Editor: Nizam Damani M.D., MBBS, MSc, FRCPI, FRCPath), due in 2006 from the International Federation of Infection Control (IFIC). The full document will be available online at IFIC's Web site: http://www.theific.org/publications.asp. NOTE: Some of these resources may appear at the end of more than one chapter, due to their applicability to more than one aspect of infection prevention and control.

Arias, K., Soule, B. (eds.): *The APIC/JCAHO Infection Control Workbook.* Washington, D.C., and Oakbrook Terrace, IL: Association for Professionals in Infection Control and Epidemiology, Inc., and Joint Commission on Accreditation of Healthcare Organizations, 2006.

Department of Health (UK): *Saving Lives: A Delivery Programme to Reduce Healthcare Associated Infections Including MRSA.* London: Department of Health, 2005. http://www.dh.gov.uk/PublicationsAndStatistics/ Publications/PublicationsLibrary/fs/en.

———: *Audit Tools for Monitoring Infection Control Standards.* London: Department of Health, 2004. http://www.dh.gov.uk/ PublicationsAndStatistics/Publications/PublicationsLibrary/fs/en.

Hospital Infection Society, Infection Control Nurses Association, Department of Health (UK): *Working Group Report. Key Indicators in Infection Control, 2004.* http://www.his.org.uk/_db/_documents/keyindicators2002-2003jan2004.pdf.

Infection Control Nurses Association: *Competencies Self-Assessment Tool.* 2001. http://www.icna.co.uk (user name and password required).

Malik R.E., Cooper R.A., Griffith C.J.: Use of audit tools to evaluate the efficacy of cleaning systems in hospitals. *Am J Infect Control* 31(3):181–187, 2003.

Society for Healthcare Epidemiology of America: An approach to the evaluation of quality indicators of the outcome of care in hospitalized patients, with a focus on nosocomial infection indicators. *Infect Control Hosp Epidemiol* 16(5):308–316, 1995. http://www.shea-online.org/publications/ shea_position_papers.cfm.

CHAPTER FOUR

Developing an Effective Infection Prevention and Control Program
Challenges, Tips, and Tools for Success

As discussed in Chapter 3, the Joint Commission International (JCI) Prevention and Control of Infections (PCI) standards place a strong emphasis on the development, implementation, and evaluation of an integrated and responsive infection prevention and control (IPC) program. Establishing such a program helps to preserve and enhance patient and staff safety and prevent adverse events.

The goal of an IPC program is to identify and reduce the risks of acquiring and transmitting infections among patients, staff, contract service workers, volunteers, students, and visitors. Effective IPC programs have many components that must work together. Several of these components will be discussed in this chapter:

- Gaining leadership support for the program
- Establishing an effective infrastructure to support the program
- Involving the whole organization in preventing infections
- Establishing the focus of the program: assessing risk and creating an IPC plan
- Designing strategies to reduce infection risk
- Developing and maintaining a continuous surveillance, data collection, and analysis process
- Evaluating the IPC program: goals, objectives, and strategies

These components, crucial to an effective program, are not always easy to achieve. This chapter identifies some of the practices and challenges associated with developing an effective IPC program and provides tips and helpful tools to help achieve success. The ideas presented here are fundamental and can be adapted for use in most care settings or organizations, depending on program management and available resources. Some of the recommendations are not required by JCI, although the relevant JCI standards are included for reference.

Gaining Leadership Support for the IPC Program

In most health care organizations, the IPC programs that receive the visible support and participation of leadership are the ones that staff members take seriously. Consequently, these programs are typically the ones that are most successful. To have an effective IPC program, leadership should be actively involved in the development, implementation, oversight, and evaluation of the program and with critical initiatives that emerge as a result of the program.[1–6]

The leaders' time is valuable and their support and presence is needed in several areas simultaneously throughout an organization. How do they devote time and energy to IPC in addition to their myriad other priorities? Several ways for leaders to actively and visibly support an IPC program are listed in Sidebar 4-1 on page 71.

An important consideration for the IPC team to gain leadership support for the IPC program is to align the IPC incentives with those of the organization and the leaders and to stress the similarities when discussing the program or proposing new activities. Increasingly leaders rely on effectiveness and efficiency when making decisions about how to allocate health care resources. In addition to delivering safe, high-quality care, they are concerned about the "bottom line" or the financial viability of the organization. The ability to demonstrate the business or financial benefits for implementing best practices in IPC will assist the IPC staff in gaining needed resources (*see* Sidebar 4-2 on page 72).

Involving Physicians in
the Infection Prevention and Control Program

It is essential to have physician leadership for the IPC program. Their expertise in the pathophysiology, prevention, and treatment of infectious diseases and knowledge of medications, vaccines, immunizations, diagnostic tests, and treatment modalities are invaluable in guiding policies and procedures that influence practices pertaining to the clinical aspects of the IPC program. Physicians who understand and partner with the IPC practitioner bring added strength to recommendations for practice changes for physicians and other clinical staff. In addition to their clinical specialty, some physicians have special training in health care epidemiology, which adds to their knowledge and expertise in leading programs of IPC, quality improvement, and patient safety.[7–10]

SIDEBAR 4-1

Methods for Supporting an
Infection Prevention and Control (IPC) Program[1,2]

- Allocate staff time and resources to the IPC program. This should include the appropriate number of IPC professionals who have the needed skills, laboratory support, technical support such as computers and printers, and administrative support such as data entry and secretarial support.
- Facilitate IPC staff access to patient records, performance improvement data, and other systems to help them complete their collection, analysis, and reporting duties.
- Provide personal protective equipment and supplies such as alcohol-based hand rubs that make it easier for staff to prevent infections.
- Attend and actively participate in meetings of the multidisciplinary IPC task force.
- Serve as a consultative resource to the IPC department as well as to any multidisciplinary teams addressing IPC issues.
- Publicly acknowledge successes in IPC such as reduced infection rates or decreased lengths of stay.
- Serve as a role model to staff (for example, use appropriate barrier techniques and sound hand hygiene practices).
- Set expectations for staff (for example, follow IPC policies, require attendance at IPC-related classes or training sessions).
- Show support for policy changes regarding IPC by supporting staff to attend in-services.
- Make timely and appropriate education and training efforts available for both clinical and nonclinical staff.
- Make compliance with IPC procedures part of performance evaluations and competency reviews.
- Coordinate IPC efforts within the community and actively communicate with public health agencies.
- Pay specific attention to addressing IPC emergencies when developing the organization's emergency management plan.
- Make IPC an overall priority for the organization.

References

1. Joint Commission Resources: *Meeting JCAHO's Infection Control Requirements: A Priority Focus Area.* Joint Commission on Accreditation of Healthcare Organizations. Oakbrook Terrace, IL: 2004.
2. Saint Thomas Hospital, Nashville, TN, USA: Methods for leadership support of infection prevention and control activities. In Arias K., Soule B. (eds.): *The APIC/JCAHO Infection Control Workbook.* Washington, D.C., and Oakbrook Terrace, IL: Association for Professionals in Infection Control and Epidemiology, Inc., and Joint Commission on Accreditation of Healthcare Organizations, 2006.

Sidebar 4-2

Clarifying the Economics of Infection Prevention and Control (IPC) Practices

IPC practices can employ simple cost-effective analyses when evaluating or proposing new or changed procedures, purchase of new devices, or additional IPC resources. A cost-effective analysis quantifies the difference between the additional health care expenditure and improved health care outcomes. This method measures how much it costs the organization to achieve an improved clinical or programmatic benefit. Some practices or procedures are more costly at the outset but save money by reducing infections. For example, using maximal sterile barriers during the insertion of central venous lines adds costs for the additional supplies but has demonstrated reduced catheter-related bloodstream infections. Antiseptic-coated urinary or vascular catheters may cost more to purchase but can prevent infections in patients with these devices. Using safety needles, which are often more expensive than regular needles, has reduced needlesticks and subsequent infections with hepatitis B and other blood-borne pathogens in health care workers.

IPC staff should be able to discuss with leaders the costs of health care–associated infections (HAIs) or outbreaks and the benefits of implementing IPC best practices. Using valid studies performed by others can serve as a benchmark. Providing this valuable information to the leaders and comparing it with the organization's experience can help leaders make resource decisions that will affect patient and staff morbidity and mortality. The same information can demonstrate the value of investing in and strengthening the IPC program as a highly cost-effective patient safety strategy. Methods for simple economic analyses can be found in several of the readings and references below.

Further Readings

The Association for Professionals in Infection Control and Epidemiology (APIC): *The Business Case for Eliminating Healthcare-Associated Infections.* Washington D.C.: APIC, in press.

Dunagan W.C., et al.: Making the business case for infection control: Pitfalls and opportunities. *Am J Infect Contro* 30:86–92, Apr. 2002.

Hu K.K., et al.: Use of maximal sterile barriers during central venous catheter insertion: Clinical and economic outcomes. *Clin Infect Dis* 39:1441–1445, Nov. 15, 2004.

French, G.: The costs of hospital infection. In French G., Friedman C. (eds.): *Infection Control: Basic Concepts and Practices,* 2nd ed. International Federation of Infection Control. 2003. http://www.theific.org/oldsite/Manual/toc.htm.

Plowman R.P., et al.: *Socioeconomic Burden of Hospital Acquired Infection.* London: Public Health Laboratory Service, 1999.

Saint, S.: Economic evaluation in infection control. In French G., Friedman C. (eds.): *Infection Control: Basic Concepts and Practices,* 2nd ed. International Federation of Infection Control. 2003. http://www.theific.org/oldsite/Manual/toc.htm.

Saint S., et al.: The potential clinical and economic benefits of silver alloy urinary catheters in preventing urinary tract infection. *Arch Intern Med* 160:2670–2675, Sep. 2000.

Veenstra D.L., Saint S., Sullivan S.D.: Cost-effectiveness of antiseptic-impregnated central venous catheters for the prevention of catheter-related bloodstream infection. *JAMA* 282:554–560, Aug. 1999.

Wilcox M.H., Dave J.: The cost of hospital-acquired infection and the value of infection control. *J Hosp Infect* 45:81–84, Jun. 2000.

To keep physicians throughout the organization interested in the IPC program, practitioners can provide them with some of the following information:

- Infection rates for surgical site infections (SSIs), ventilator-associated pneumonia (VAP), bloodstream infections, and urinary tract infections (UTIs)
- Antibiograms indicating the organization's rates of multidrug-resistant organisms such as methicillin-resistant *Staphylococcus aureus* (MRSA) vancomycin-resistant enterococci (VRE), and other resistant organisms such as *Acinetobacter baumanii*
- New or proposed policies that will affect physician practice. It is important to involve them in the development of these policies.
- Updated scientific information and new evidence-based guidelines
- Governmental documents and regulations related to IPC
- For surgeons, specific SSI rates

IPC Staff as Leaders

Although strong administrative and physician leadership involvement is crucial to the success of any IPC program (PCI.6), dedicated IPC professionals are needed to manage the day-to-day operations of the program, identify areas of improvement, and help address any issues that arise. The responsibilities of this individual or individuals are numerous and include the following:

- *Risk assessment*—continual evaluation of infection risks by both formal and informal means using quantitative or qualitative methods and including key personnel
- *Surveillance and investigation*—including surveillance system planning and design, data collection, investigation, interpretation, and communication regarding findings
- *Prevention*—including helping develop IPC policies and procedures and IPC strategies for such areas as hand hygiene, equipment cleaning, disinfection and sterilization, and hazardous waste collection and management
- *Research*—including staying abreast of national guidelines, laws, and clinical pathways addressing IPC and researching new and emerging diseases
- *Education and training*—including all staff training and education on IPC issues. Education efforts might start with the assessment of staff needs and involve training programs, frequent communication, and evaluation.
- *Response*—responding to infection clusters, an outbreak, pandemic, or bioterrorist event. To prepare for such events, this individual should be knowledgeable about cluster and outbreak

investigation methods and be involved in emergency planning efforts and drills.

- *Management*—running the day-to-day operations of the IPC program. This could include program evaluation, regulatory compliance, reporting, and planning for current and future projects.
- *Consulting*—working with staff to address IPC questions and solve problems and collaborating with other departments on policies and procedures (for example, appropriate isolation of patients with communicable diseases and product selection for patient care). Also includes input on the care of the environment and construction projects to ensure that staff consider infection prevention issues, such as room and floor layout, water system and air flow design, supply access, hand-washing facilities, and appropriate isolation and quarantine facilities.[11]

Establishing an Effective Infrastructure for the IPC Program

How do organizations make sure that IPC programs function effectively and address all the necessary issues? One way is to establish an infrastructure that supports the systems and functions of the program. This can be challenging in countries with limited resources. There are several essential components of a strong infrastructure.[12–15]

Creating a Multidisciplinary Team to Oversee the IPC Program

One of the primary structural elements of an IPC program is a multidisciplinary IPC team, task force, or formal committee that is charged with creating, implementing, and monitoring the IPC program. JCI does not specifically require the creation of a multidisciplinary committee, but suggests that this is one method to oversee and coordinate the program (PCI.7). A multidisciplinary committee brings together the perspectives of persons who implement IPC in their respective departments or services. Their experiences add richness and reality to the program. Some organizations exist in states or countries where licensure law, rules, or regulations specify that a formal infection control (IC) committee be assigned to the IPC function.

A multidisciplinary IPC group, committee, or team should be broadly inclusive of related departments and major clinical service areas (which, in some cases, may be only medicine and nursing). The group should include some of the following representatives:

- Administration
- Central sterile processing
- Environmental services/housekeeping personnel
- Equipment maintenance personnel (biomedical engineering staff)

- Facilities management, including engineering and maintenance personnel
- Information management staff
- Laboratory personnel, particularly microbiology
- Medical staff (for example, department heads or representatives of surgery, pediatrics, medicine, emergency services)
- Nursing leaders and staff
- Patient safety/performance improvement specialists
- Pharmacists

The team should meet regularly and, ideally, there should be active participation, an agenda of topics, reports or policies, action items, action steps with time frames, and identification of responsible parties. The organization should provide education and training in IPC for the team members, as well as clarity about their roles and responsibilities.

The first responsibility of this team will be to establish the focus of the organization's IPC program by assessing and analyzing the risks specific to the organization. Following the risk assessment, the team should develop a well-defined and specific IPC plan that includes goals and objectives to reduce infection risks.

As part of the infrastructure that nurtures and supports the IPC program, there should be clear, strong connections between IPC, quality improvement, and patient safety. For optimal function, the infection control process is integrated with the organization's overall program for quality improvement and patient safety (PCI.11).[16,17] In those organizations with a quality improvement committee, IPC plans should be reviewed with the committee to obtain feedback and suggestions for improvement and to integrate IPC data with other quality and patient safety data. This will enhance the use of all the information for the best decision-making process to improve or maintain patient care and staff safety.

Program Management

In addition to a multidisciplinary team, such as an IPC committee or IPC advisory council, organizations should designate an individual who has experience with IPC to take the lead in creating and managing the program. He or she should be trained in IPC or have the opportunity to be mentored and coached by an experienced person or persons. The individual should seek feedback from other areas of the organization during the development of the IPC program, such as the nursing, respiratory therapy, and pharmacy staff. The person who accepts the lead responsibility to coordinate the program will have responsibilities that include working with the IC committee or others to set criteria for defining HAIs and for establishing the surveillance process and methods for collecting, analyzing, and reporting data to the appropriate persons and committees. The lead IC physician is also responsible for communicating with all parts of the organization to make certain that the program is ongoing and proactive (PCI.7). Regardless of who leads the daily IPC activities, it is essential to have representatives from at least medicine and nursing involved in the oversight of the IPC program (PCI.8). The statistician, data collection staff, central sterilization manager, microbiology, pharmacy, or operating theater supervisor can also provide valuable input. As discussed with the IC committee, who the participants in the oversight group will be depends on the size and services of the organization.

IPC Staff

To have the appropriate number and skill mix of IPC professionals, organizations should take into consideration the following factors:

- The scope of the IPC program, including the type and services the organization provides. Organizations providing multiple services (such as hospitals with laboratories) need to design IPC departments or services that meet the needs of both areas.
- The characteristics of patient populations. Different patient populations have varying needs regarding IPC. For example, immunocompromised populations are at higher risk for infection, and those organizations that serve a predominantly immunocompromised population need to factor in those risks when designing an IPC department.
- Economic pressures. Although the ideal staff of IPC professionals might not be economically feasible for some organizations, an effort should be made to address the needs of the organization within the budget available. Some creative ways to do this can include time sharing and resource sharing with other organizations in the community.
- Demographics of the workforce. If a health care organization has a significant number of employees for whom English is not the first language, special attention should be given to make sure that IPC staff is able to communicate effectively with staff and patients about IPC issues.
- Responsibilities of the IPC professional and the number of occupied beds that he or she oversees for infection issues.[18]

One method used to expand the IPC resources is the Link Nurse Program that is prevalent in the UK and other countries. A similar approach is the Nurse Liaison Program used in some U.S. hospitals. For both of these methods, staff nurses who are selected or volunteer are provided basic training in IPC and take a leadership role on their units. They become the extended arms of the IPC practitioner and may do limited surveillance, help develop policies and procedures, observe practices, and take on other responsibilities.[19–23]

IPC professionals should have basic knowledge of IPC theories, as well as skills and abilities that would enable them to perform their responsibilities to implement and maintain an effective IPC program. There are several ways for IPC professionals to obtain knowledge and skills, including formal training, informal on-the-job mentoring, experience with managing IPC challenges, and working toward and obtaining IPC certification. Currently the UK offers a diploma to IPC practitioner, IC physicians, microbiologists, epidemiologists, and others who complete the requirements of training.[25] The Certification Board of Infection Control (CBIC) in the United States offers the certification examination (based on the U.S. practice analysis) in many countries to these same professionals.[24,25,26]

After the appropriate number and skill mix of staff are determined, organizations should make sure that all IPC professionals are adequately trained and that their competency is verified routinely. These individuals should know the underlying principles of IPC and be educated on or have job experience in areas of applying epidemiological principles to prevent infections. The successful completion of a course in IPC or IPC professional certification might be a benchmark for competence in this area.

Policies and Procedures

Policies and procedures are part of the infrastructure for the IPC program. Clear policies that incorporate the basic principles and concepts of IPC provide guidance for patient care, health care worker safety, care of the environment, and management of IPC emergencies. Maintaining current policies that are based on scientific evidence is essential. The policies should be disseminated to all appropriate staff who should receive education to ensure that they understand the policies and can perform the procedures. Periodically, selected policies and procedures are monitored or audited to determine if they are effective and if staff is complying. Both process and outcome monitoring are useful. These methods are discussed in the section "Identifying Risks Through Surveillance, Data Collection, and Analysis" beginning on page 96.

Involving the Whole Organization

The risk of infection occurs throughout a health care organization, and any program designed to prevent and control infection must involve *all* areas of an organization to be effective. Several of the PCI standards guide organizations to use an integrated approach to IPC, including PCI.1, .7, and .11 (*see* Chapter 2).

IPC Policies and Procedures That Apply to All Staff

The policies for hand hygiene, barrier precautions and isolation measures, reprocessing or reusing supplies, immunizations or health screenings for staff, and safe needle use apply to all personnel. These policies should be developed by the IPC staff in partnership with the person(s) who will implement or is affected by the policy directives. Service-specific policies help to incorporate appropriate IPC practices in the daily operations of various parts of the organization, such as the operating theater, radiology, pharmacy, and other key services.

Educating and Communicating with Staff

Education and communication promote IPC as an organizationwide program. Education leading to behavioral change can be a powerful deterrent to spreading HAI. Each individual affiliated with a health care organization must understand his or her role in IPC efforts. To accomplish this, organizations must continually educate staff areas about the following topics:

- How infections are transmitted in the health care setting; both to patients and to staff
- The role of health care providers in preventing and controlling infection transmission, including their role in providing leadership, direct care, or supportive services
- How health care providers can identify problems or potential problems related to IPC and the policies to address those problems
- How to report identified problems, including the information to report and where to report them
- How caregivers can preserve their health to help preserve the safety of their patients (*see* the Case Scenario beginning on page 79)

Although most organizations teach precautions for staff members who provide direct care, they sometimes overlook staff who might be exposed to and act as carriers of infection. In addition to the direct care clinical staff, other persons who interact with patients or might have contact with patients or their environment, equipment, or wastes include biomedical technicians, facilities staff, waste and garbage handlers, plumbers, electricians, delivery personnel, personal aides, and housekeepers.

Direct care staff should know how to identify risk factors for infection in its patient populations. The elderly—many of whom might suffer from chronic illnesses, lack of mobility, and immunodeficiency—are particularly vulnerable and may show few symptoms in the presence of infection. Evaluating subtle signs should be part of the skill set of those who care for this population. Patients with indwelling devices such as urinary, peripheral, or central venous catheters and those undergoing invasive therapy, ventilator support, and dialysis are considered high-risk populations, as is anyone undergoing surgery or other invasive procedures. Staff members who care for these patients or the equipment used to determine diagnosis or administer therapy should receive education that focuses on the particular risks of the care processes and the devices. Thus, in an organizationwide IPC program, education must address the basic core principles of IPC and be designed specifically for certain populations, procedures, or pathogens.

CASE SCENARIO

Using Education to Change Staff Perception of the Importance of Vaccinations

A large ambulatory clinic had an organizationwide, comprehensive, voluntary program to control exposure to tuberculosis and hepatitis B (HBV) infections in health care workers. Staff members were strongly encouraged to take the HBV vaccine, but could decline. The infection prevention and control (IPC) practitioner at the clinic believed that increasing numbers of new staff were beginning to decline HBV vaccination, although the declination rate was not being tracked. The IPC practitioner decided to keep a record of the number of staff members who chose to decline HBV immunization over six months. As suspected, the declination rate was increasing each month as new staff, employees, and contract employees went through the orientation process.

The IPC practitioner developed an interview form, and each new staff member who declined HBV immunization was asked to share his or her reasons. Very quickly, a common theme emerged—there was widespread misinformation regarding catching the disease from the vaccine. An educational intervention was developed and implemented to communicate the facts about live and synthetic vaccines and to increase acceptance of HBV immunization. The clinic's IPC and employee health committee was made aware of the improvements achieved in reducing the declination rate. The Infection Control Committee recommended that the practitioner continue monitoring for the next six months to ensure that the educational intervention was still effective.

Education for staff should include an initial orientation, annual IPC updates, and periodic information about new policies or recent developments such as emerging diseases, resistant organisms, or new methods to prevent infection. It is important for IPC staff to assess the educational needs of health care workers, use varied teaching and learning methods, and evaluate whether learning has taken place from the educational offering (*see* Chapter 5).

Communication with Staff

In addition to providing education, organizations must communicate to all physicians, nurses, other clinical and support staff, students, and volunteers the IPC goals, objectives, and initiatives and share results of any performance improvement projects under way. Staff and leaders must have the most current information so they can apply it to their practice in caring for patients, protecting themselves from acquiring infection, or guiding the work of the organization.

It is also important to communicate IPC information to the committees that govern the organization, such as the administrative committee, medical and nursing committees, governing board, and committees that oversee the organization's environment and facilities. As patients move from one part of the hospital to another or from the hospital to the outpatient or ambulatory care setting, it is essential for their well-being and to prevent gaps in therapies to communicate any IPC information to the next level of care. Organizations should develop systems to ensure that this communication occurs. IPC practitioners, nurses, care managers, discharge coordinators, and others can participate.

Providing staff with information about how a particular initiative has improved safety and reduced infections can go a long way toward ensuring compliance throughout the organization. Good venues for communicating such information to staff include group in-services or one-to-one conversations, newsletters, staff meetings, intranet sites, videos, and break-room bulletin boards.

Communication of Infection Prevention and Control Data and Information to Families and Visitors

In many settings, the patient's family and other visitors are an integral part of the patient's care. They participate in hygiene and daily activities, wound care, ambulation of the patient, and other direct care activities. In some settings the parents are the primary caregivers for pediatric or adult patients. In addition, the family and visitors may bring meals to the patient and even prepare them at the hospital or clinic. Thus, it is essential that the family be included in the communication program about infection prevention methods to help them best care for their family member and to protect themselves and others from acquiring or transmitting infection.

Participating in Organizationwide Committees

Committees outside of IPC often make decisions that influence IPC practices. In an organizationwide IPC program, IPC personnel should serve on the committees that develop policies and procedures affecting the care of patients or the well-being of staff as related to IPC. This might include quality improvement, patient safety, construction, product selection, or other activities. Sending communications from the IC committee to other committees and to the staff is another method for coordinating and integrating the IPC program throughout the organization.

Building Relationships Within the Organization

Dedicated IPC practitioners to oversee everyday operations of an IPC program, along with a physician dedicated to IPC, are key to the operation of

SIDEBAR 4-3

IPC-Related Process Measures

These measures have been suggested, along with others, for inclusion in the current revision of U.S. Centers for Disease Prevention and Control patient isolation guidelines, which are still under review:

- Provision of education and training via orientation and/or annual in-service education to 95% of employed patient care staff
- Standardized observational studies comparing required compliance with standard precautions versus observed compliance (applied to selected high-risk areas or processes at least annually)
- Assessment of availability and accessibility of alcohol-based hand hygiene products
- Use of health care–associated infection data to identify potential patient-to-patient transmission of infectious agents and multidrug-resistant organisms

Source: Adapted from Strausbaugh L., et al., and the Centers for Disease Control and Prevention Healthcare Infection Control Practices Advisory Committee: *Guidelines to Prevent Transmission of Infectious Agents in Healthcare Settings 2002*. Draft #2, Feb. 15, 2002.

the program. However, these professionals are only part of the IPC process. Successful IPC programs are a product of many individuals throughout a health care organization working together to prevent the spread of infection (PCI.8). IPC professionals should identify key people throughout the organization and in the community and communicate frequently with them about IPC activities. These key people might represent the following areas:

- Administration (including data collection expert, statistician, central sterilization manager, operating theater supervisor)
- Clinical/medical staff (including epidemiologist, microbiologist)
- Facility management
- Housekeeping
- Nursing
- Pharmacy
- Public health (*see* Sidebar 4-3 above)

Creating Multidisciplinary Performance Improvement Teams

When vulnerabilities in IPC practice are identified, and system issues become apparent, the organization should initiate improvement projects that will result in better care for the patients, safer work environments for staff, and reduced risk for families and visitors. When the issue crosses several departments or services or more than one type of care setting, the most effective way to address these issues is with a multidisciplinary team that melds the experience and expertise of all those involved. It is important to include on these teams those persons who truly understand the work setting or the technical aspects of the facility. They will be most knowledgeable about the current practices and the barriers in the workplace and can provide valuable input to solutions for improvements. For broader issues that cross several care settings or many organizations, a network of professionals can work as a team.[27–29]

Establishing the Focus of the Infection Prevention and Control Program

Performing the Risk Assessment and Creating an IPC Plan

Standards PCI.1 and PCI.2 state that the IPC program must address IPC issues that are epidemiologically important to the organization, including important infections, infection sites, and associated devices. This information is used to establish priorities and activities to prevent and reduce the incidence of HAIs. PCI.3 states that the organization identifies the procedures and processes associated with the risk of infection and implements strategies to reduce infection risk. It is thus important for an organization to review those processes and, as appropriate, implement policies, procedures, education, improvement, and other activities to reduce risk of infection. Together these three standards convey a strong message that the organization will be expected to perform some type of risk assessment to determine the priorities of the IPC program.[30,31]

Performing a risk assessment should be one of the first activities of a new IPC program and an ongoing activity of established programs. Optimally, the risk assessment and refocusing of program activities should be performed at least annually and more often if needed due to changes in circumstances, such as the addition of a new service or a change in population or community events.

A risk assessment is a careful examination of events that could cause infections, harm, or even death to patients, staff, families, or visitors to the facility. The plan that evolves from the assessment identifies methods to minimize, mitigate, or manage risks that might occur.

The risk assessment process includes an analysis of existing information—such as surveillance data, injuries, or other reports of adverse events—resource limitations, and information that can be gathered proactively through surveys or focus groups of staff or a review of the scientific literature. Some risks may be anticipated based on environmental changes, emerging diseases, or events in other health care settings or in the world. For example, in each country there are differences in emerging or reemerging infections that affect both community and hospital populations (*see* Chapter 1). Some conditions, such as the potential for an avian influenza pandemic, are a risk for which every health care organization in the world should prepare. Natural disasters may be anticipated based on a country's location and climate. There are also different economic realities for health care organizations, depending on the country in which the organization is located. One model for evaluating infection risks based on economic pressures is presented in Sidebar 4-4 on page 84.

General topics or categories that can be considered in a risk assessment include, but are not limited to, the following:

- Characteristics of the patient populations served by the health care facility
- Geography, community, and environmental setting of the health care organization
- Type of care, treatment, and services provided
- Patient care and facility environment
- Locally adopted clinical pathways or practice guidelines
- Risks to health care workers
- Emergencies affecting the health care settings
- Current local, state, and federal laws
- Results of past studies, surveillance data, audits, or clinical findings
- Information from the World Health Organization (WHO), ministries of health, U.S. Centers for Disease Control and Prevention (US CDC) and other public health agencies

Each organization can select its own methodology for performing a risk assessment. One method is to establish general categories of risk such as high-risk or high-incidence health care infections, the characteristics of the geographic setting of the organization, potential natural disasters, emergency preparedness, risks to health care workers, and the distinct attributes of the major populations cared for by the organization.

After the general categories have been determined, the organization can identify and analyze specific risk events in each category. For example, one category might be risks to health care workers, and the individual risk events may include sharps injuries, exposure to tuberculosis (TB) or other communicable disease, or degree of compliance with hand hygiene or iso-lation procedures. Another category might be high-risk infections and include specific risk events such as catheter-related bloodstream infections, ventillator-associated pneumonia (VAP), and post–C-section endometritis. Each of these specific potential risk events is assessed as part of the overall risk analysis (*see* Table 4-1 on page 86).

The two basic questions one asks to assess risk are (1) How likely is it that a risk event will occur? and (2) How severe would the risk event be should it occur? For deeper analysis, additional questions can also be posed. A list of potential risk assessment queries is found in Sidebar 4-5 on page 85.

The process for completing a risk assessment includes several steps, as indicated in Figure 4-1 on page 86.

SIDEBAR 4-4

Characteristics of Hospitals

Hospitals and clinics around the world reflect the economic realities of their locations. It is important to consider these when assessing infection risk, planning for infection prevention and control (IPC) activities, and evaluating available resources. A model for considering which "tier" best reflects an organization's risks is presented below. All tiers may exist simultaneously in a given country.

Tier 1

In Tier 1 hospitals adequate supplies of clean water, sterile instruments and supplies for contact with normally sterile body sites, and clean equipment and supplies for contact with mucous membranes and nonintact skin are rarely available. Open versus closed systems are often used for intravascular devices, fluids for ventilation, and urinary drainage. Facilities may prepare their own fluids for infusion and irrigation. Adequate hand hygiene is challenging. In Tier 1 hospitals patients often share beds and supplies, and families often provide food and such supplies as syringes and medications and administer much of the care, particularly for children. These facilities may have little infection prevention information or a minimal IPC program and can have frequent outbreaks of health care–associated infections (HAIs) because of unsterile fluids, instruments, and supplies. Employee training in infection prevention is highly variable and often nominal. Procedures such as transfusions and injection safety may facilitate transmission of infections, such as HIV and hepatitis.[1] In this tier, maternal-child infections contribute disproportionately to morbidity and mortality. Neonatal mortality rates (deaths in the first 28 days of life) are as high as 40 to 50 per 1,000 live births in many of the poorest parts of the world.[2]

Tier 2

Tier 2 hospitals reflect better economic conditions. Hospitals in this group generally have access to clean water and have sterilizers and cleaning processes, but the availability of sterile or high-level disinfected instruments, medications, and supplies is variable. Employees have more training in IPC and IPC information is more available than in Tier 1 hospitals. A formal IPC program may exist, with responsibilities assigned to a committee and/or individuals. Patients are housed in large wards and intensive care units (ICUs); private rooms are scarce. Some open systems may be used for IV fluids, respiratory care, and urinary drainage. Quality standards are increased in this tier and, in some cases, are measured. Hand hygiene occurs with hand washing or alcohol rubs.

Tier 3

Tier 3 hospitals have single-use sterile instruments and supplies, adequate reprocessing techniques, and abundant clean water. Closed systems are used for drainage of fluids, reducing infection risk. Significant attention is paid to the cleanliness and comfort of the patients, who often have private rooms. Most facilities have formal IPC programs with IPC committees. Education of staff and certification of individual knowledge and practices exists and may be required. Complex sur-

SIDEBAR 4-4—CONTINUED

veillance systems demonstrate transmission of infectious agents among the patients, particularly in ICUs. Outbreaks of HAIs are rare and quickly recognized. Guidelines and equipment are available, but even in this tier compliance with recommendations for hand hygiene, presurgical antibiotic prophylaxis, and insertion and maintenance of invasive devices such as central vascular lines and ventilators may not follow evidence-based guidelines.

References

1. Hauri A.M., Armstrong G.L., Hutin Y.J.: The global burden of disease attributable to contaminated injections given in health care settings. *Int J STD AIDS* 15:7–16, Jan. 2004.
2. Zaidi A.K., et al.: Hospital-acquired neonatal infections in developing countries. *Lancet* 365:1175–1188, Apr. 2005.

Source: Patricia Lynch, R.N., M.B.A., Chair, International Federation of Infection Control. Used with permission.

SIDEBAR 4-5

Questions to Analyze Potential Infection Risk Events

- What are the potential or actual risks that may lead to infections in this organization?
- What is the probability that any given risk event will occur?
- If the risk event occurs, how severe could it be?
- How frequently might the risk event occur?
- What is the organization's ability to identify the risk?
- What is the scope of response that would be required by the organization to reduce or eliminate the risk?
- How prepared is the organization at this time?
- How prepared is the organization to respond?
- How well does leadership support response to the event?

Source: Adapted from Soule B.: Analyzing risk and setting goals and objectives for the infection control program. In Arias K., Soule B. (eds.): *The APIC/JCAHO Infection Control Workbook*. Washington, D.C., and Oakbrook Terrace, IL: Association for Professionals in Infection Control and Epidemiology, Inc., and Joint Commission on Accreditation of Healthcare Organizations, 2006, p. 49.

TABLE 4-1

Risk Categories and Risk Factors for Infection Prevention and Control

Risk Category	Risk Factors

Geographic location	Natural disasters
	    Tornadoes, floods, hurricanes, earthquakes
	Breakdown or absence of municipal services
	Broken water main, contaminated water supply,
	    strike or work stoppage by sanitation employees
	Accidents in the community
	    Mass transit (airplane, train, bus)
	Fires involving mass casualties
	Intentional acts—Bioterrorism, "Dirty Bomb"
	    Contamination of food and water supplies
	Prevalence of disease linked with vectors, temperature,
	    other environmental factors

Community	Community outbreaks of transmissible infectious
	    diseases (influenza, meningitis)
	Diseases linked to food and water contamination
	    (for example, salmonella, hepatitis A)
	Vaccine-preventable illness in unvaccinated population
	Infections associated with immigrant or
	    migrant populations in geographic area
	Public health infrastructure
	Socioeconomic levels
	    (for example, income and education)

Organization programs and services	Cardiac service Orthopedic service Neonatology Dialysis Long term care Ambulatory clinics Hospice (end of life care) Home care Behavioral health care
Special populations served	Women and children Frail elderly Behavioral health care Long term care Rehabilitation Diseases associated with lifestyle Predisposition for illnesses resulting from cognitive and physical changes Migratory populations
High-risk patients	Surgical Intensive care unit Neonatal or Pediatric intensive care unit Oncology Dialysis Transplant Rehabilitation

TABLE 4-1—CONTINUED

Risk Category	Risk Factors
Health care worker risks	Understanding disease transmission and prevention Degree of compliance with infection prevention techniques and policies—hand hygiene Use of personal protective equipment and isolation Sharps injuries Screening for transmissible diseases Work restriction guidelines Practice accountability issues
Medical procedures	Invasiveness of procedure Equipment used for procedure Knowledge and technical expertise of those performing procedure Adequate preparation of patient Adherence to recommended infection prevention techniques
Equipment and devices	Cleaning, disinfection, transport, and storage for intravenous (IV) pumps, suction equipment, other equipment Sterilization or disinfection process for scopes, surgical instruments, prostheses Complexity of device Skill and experience of user Safety features: user dependent or automatic Reuse of single-use devices Preparation of IV fluids or medications Open versus closed systems
Environmental issues	Construction, renovation, alterations Utilities performance Environmental cleanliness and safety
Emergency preparedness	Staff education Managing influx of infectious patients Triaging patients Isolation, barriers, personal protective equipment Utilities and supplies Security
Resource limitations	Staffing limitations for nursing, physicians, clinical support staff, other support staff, environmental services, infection prevention and control professionals Sterile supplies Congested patient care areas
Organization's surveillance data	Catheter-related bloodstream infections Ventilator-associated pneumonia Catheter-associated urinary tract infections Surgical site infections Gastrointestinal infections Sepsis Other

Source: Adapted from Soule B.: Analyzing risk and setting goals and objectives for the infection control Program. In Arias K., Soule B. (eds.): *The APIC/JCAHO Infection Control Workbook*. Washington, D.C., and Oakbrook Terrace, IL: Association for Professionals in Infection Control and Epidemiology, Inc., and Joint Commission on Accreditation of Healthcare Organizations, 2006, pp. 50–52.

FIGURE 4-1

The Risk Assessment Process

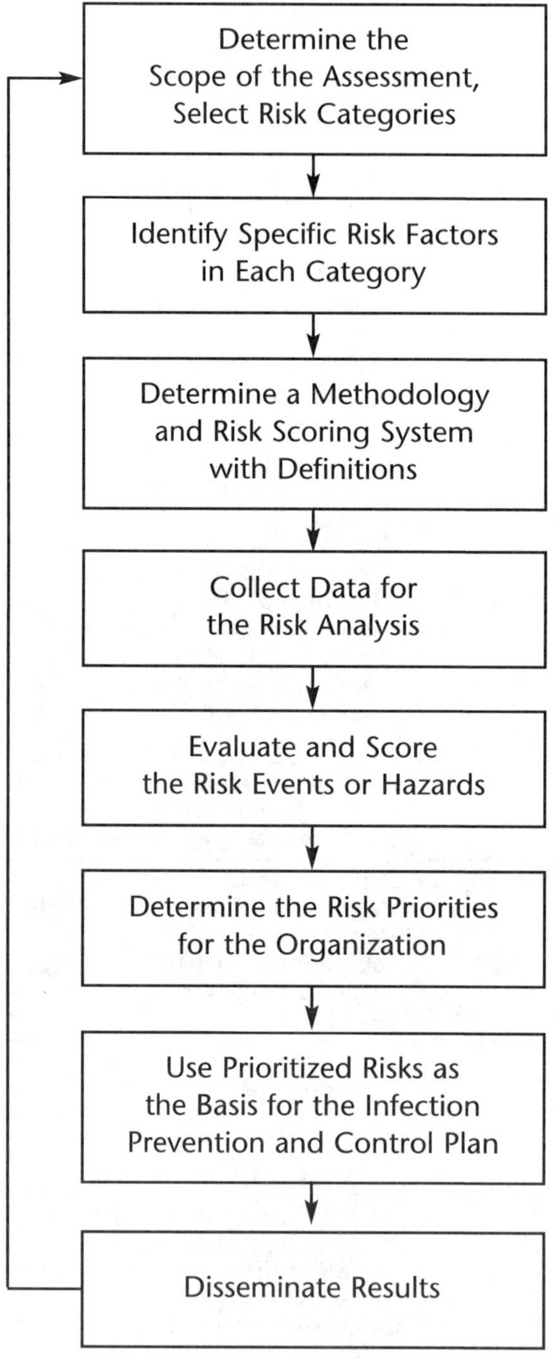

Source: Adapted from Soule B.: Analyzing risk and setting goals and objectives for the infection control program. In Arias K., Soule B. (eds.): *The APIC/JCAHO Infection Control Workbook.* Washington, D.C., and Oakbrook Terrace, IL: Association for Professionals in Infection Control and Epidemiology, Inc., and Joint Commission on Accreditation of Healthcare Organizations, 2006, p. 47.

The risk analysis process should be systematic and include at least those persons who are responsible for the IPC program and others who are key leaders or staff who support the program. Adequate time should be allotted to gather data to assess risk events. The IPC team may need information from medical records, finance, special services, or the public health agency in addition to surveillance data.

The method for performing the risk assessment can be quantitative, using numerical values to rate the risk events, or it can be qualitative, using written processes to discuss the risks and their potential harm.[30,32] Either method will be useful if the persons who are participating and those who will receive the report understand it. *See* Figure 4-2 on page 90 for qualitative description of risks and priorities.

When the analysis is completed, the risks considered the highest priority for the organization are selected and presented to the IC committee and administration for approval and support. After the leadership agrees to the selected priorities, they should support the work with the needed resources. In some countries and organizations, there may not be additional infrastructure or monetary resources for all priorities. For those, leaders can make the issues highly visible and convey their importance to the organization and staff and ensure that there are clear policies and procedures, education, and monitoring or auditing to make changes where possible. More steps and details of the risk assessment can be found in Table 4-2 on page 92.

Developing the Infection Prevention and Control Plan

After the IPC priorities have been approved, the organization uses them to develop the IPC plan. The plan has two main parts: (1) the background information about the program and services offered by the IPC department, and (2) the action plan for the year.

Background Information

For background information, the plan might contain the purpose or mission of the IPC program and the vision or future of the program. For example, the mission might state: "The infection prevention and control program minimizes risk of infection to promote a high quality of care, safety, and well-being in patients, staff, and visitors." The IPC plan may include information about the infrastructure of the program, including the number of staff and their roles; the IC committee; how medicine, nursing, and others participate in coordinating the program (PCI.8); and the authority of designated individuals (for example, chairman, IC physician, IC nurse, or administrator) to make IPC decisions for actions such as placing a patient in isolation, closing a unit, or stopping surgery because of infection risks. The plan may discuss the scope of services that the IPC team offers to the organization, including education, surveillance and

FIGURE 4-2

Infection Prevention and Control Risk Assessment

Population at Risk	Indicator or Activity	Method of Analysis and Target	Rationale	Priority			
				Risk of occurring	Impact on patient	Prevention potential	Overall priority
Adult Intensive Care Units (ICUs), Medical Intensive Care Unit (MICU)/ Critical Care Unit (CCU), Surgical Intensive Care Unit (SICU), Neonatal Intensive Care Unit (NICU), Burn Intensive Care Unit (BICU)	**Outcome indicator:** Ventilator-associated pneumonia (VAP)	**Rates:** VAP per 1,000 ventilator days. Compare to National Healthcare Safety Network (NHSN) or National Nosocomial Infections Surveillance System (NNIS) data for same type ICU. **Target:** 25th–50th percentile for NHSN or NNIS	Ventilators are associated with an increased risk of pneumonia.	MICU, CCU: moderate NICU, SICU: high BICU: high	Serious infection Serious infection Serious infection	Moderately preventable Moderately preventable Somewhat preventable	**Moderate** **Moderate** **Moderate**
Neonatal Intensive Care (NICU)	**Outcome indicator:** Epidemiologically significant organisms (methicillin-resistant *Staphylococcus aureus* [MRSA], resistant gram negatives, all Serratia, and unusual organisms with a possible environmental source). Antibiogram for hospital-associated MRSA	Calculate rates per 1,000 patient days. Compare to historical data. Monitor for trends and develop targets for reduction as necessary.	Prevention of epidemics requires prompt interventions when increases in rates are identified or when serious infections due to unusual (possibly environmental) organisms are identified.	Patients are at higher risk of infection from both MRSA and opportunistic organisms. Risk of clusters is higher in ICUs; (intensity of contact)	Depends on colonization vs. infection. Isolation (psychological impact and cost) is also a factor.	Routine infection control measures and isolation may interrupt transmission. Risks from environment not always apparent.	**High**
	Outcome indicator: Central line associated–bloodstream infection	Calculate rates per 1,000 central line days, stratified by birth weight. Compare to NHSN or NNIS data. **Target:** 50th percentile	Central lines are associated with an increased risk of bloodstream infection.	Low to moderate	Potentially severe	Moderately preventable	**High**

FIGURE 4-2—CONTINUED

Population at Risk	Indicator or Activity	Method of Analysis and Target	Rationale	Priority			
				Risk of occurring	Impact on patient	Prevention potential	Overall priority
Surgical Patients	**Outcome indicator:** Surgical site infections (SSIs) for selected procedures (abdominal hysterectomy, vaginal hysterectomy, hip prosthesis, knee prosthesis, cardiac surgery, non–Coronary Artery Bypass Graft [CABG], vascular procedures, colon surgery).	Calculate precentage of SSIs per procedure, stratified by NNIS risk index. **Target:** 50th percentile for procedure compared to NNIS	Surgical patients are at risk of infection. Risk factors may be analyzed and interventions planned to improve outcome.	Depends upon procedure	All SSIs are potentially serious, possibly resulting in additional procedures.	Moderately preventable	**Moderate**
	Process indicator: Antibiotic prophylaxis	Compare to Surgical Infection Prevention (SIP) data as a benchmark for selection of agent, timing (< 1 hr before incision)	Antibiotic prophylaxis is an important factor in preventing SSI.	Low to moderate risk of timing or selection not within parameters	Potentially serious	High: prophylaxis an important factor in preventing SSI	**High**
Employees	**Outcome indicator:** Needlestick prevention	Report number and trends, with attention to type of needle and blood-borne pathogen exposure. Report number of conversions. **Target:** 20% reduction	Needlesticks pose a significant risk for health care personnel.	High number of sticks and sharps injuries	Low conversion rate, but worrisome and costly	Preventable when safety sharps are available	**High**

Source: Parkland Health & Hospital System, Dallas, TX, USA. Used with permission.

Table 4-2

Steps in Performing a Risk Assessment

Steps	Details
Form a multidisciplinary group to perform the risk assessment.	Engage IPC practitioners, physicians, nursing, support staff, leaders, others.
Determine the general categories of risks to be addressed.	Consider risks internal to the organization and those that are external; risks that are known and those that can be anticipated.
Identify the specific risk events in each category.	Develop a list of risk events or risk factors in each category.
Select a method for the analysis (in other words, quantitative or qualitative).	Develop a format and template to support the method selected.
Select a scoring system.	Use numerical ratings or "High, Medium, or Low," or other. Define numbers or terms.
Collect the information needed to assess each risk event.	Obtain information from the following: Surveillance data Medical records Financial information Accidents and incidents Deaths Other
Score each potential risk event using predetermined criteria or definitions.	See above.
Select the highest risks for the organization as the priorities.	Determine which risks pose the greatest threat of harm to patients, staff, others.
	Work with multidisciplinary group to make the determinations.
Obtain approval from leadership.	Present priorities to the IC committee for formal approval. Also seek approval from organizational leaders.
Develop the IPC plan using the risk priorities.	Use the priorities to develop goals, measurable objectives, and evaluation plan.
Disseminate results and IPC plan.	Distribute to leadership, clinical units, service or department heads, key staff, others.

Source: Adapted from Arias K., Soule B. (eds.): *The APIC/JCAHO Infection Control Workbook.* Washington, D.C., and Oakbrook Terrace, IL: Association for Professionals in Infection Control and Epidemiology, Inc., and Joint Commission on Accreditation of Healthcare Organizations, 2006.

outbreak investigation, developing policies and procedures, overseeing the environment and medical equipment, and consulting with staff throughout the hospital for IPC problems. The integration of the IPC program with quality improvement and patient safety (PCI.11) and the education offered to staff and others (PCI.12) are also appropriate topics for the IPC plan. The plan may address the availability and appropriate use of gloves, masks, soap, and disinfectants (PCI.4); what surveillance cultures will be collected; and the training of the staff that collect the specimens (PCI.5). The plan may also explain how the IPC program uses current scientific knowledge, accepted practice guidelines, and applicable law and regulation (PCI.9) to guide activities and policies. IPC's relationship with the quality improvement and patient safety programs are also appropriate topics (PCI.11).

Annual Action Plan
The second and most important part of the IPC plan is the section that describes the priorities, goals, objectives, and evaluation process. This is also where the organization identifies the strategies to reduce infection risk (PCI.3) that evolve from the risk priorities, goals, and objectives. The key to having a useful and dynamic plan is to keep it simple and to state clearly how strategies will be accomplished and measured. The grid in Table 4-3 on page 94 provides one example for capturing the key elements of the IPC plan in a way that is easy to monitor, update, and describe. Using a grid like this can also provide a tool for teaching, describing, and marketing the program to the organization and external agencies, as well as for developing reports. The example shown in Table 4-3 is one method.

Implementing Strategies to Reduce Infection Risk

The IPC team develops risk reduction strategies on an ongoing basis. Some strategies are short term. They are developed, based on surveillance data, in response to consultations with the staff or during observations of the environment or care practices made on rounds. Some interventions evolve from known areas of risk based on literature and research and the experience of other IPC programs. Adverse outcomes may also stimulate new strategies or indicate the need for change in other areas. Standard PCI.3 provides a list of processes associated with infection risk where JCI expects organizations to implement risk reduction strategies.

At least annually, as the organization establishes the focus of the IPC program, the IPC team develops more long-term intervention strategies based on the risk assessment and the goals and objectives that have been selected for that year. It is important that the most effective strategies are initiated. Several tactics can help IPC practitioners choose the most

TABLE 4-3

Sample Hospital Infection Control Plan

Risk Priority	Organizational Goal	Infection Control Goal	Measurable Objective	Method(s)	Evaluation	Participants
High ventilator-associated pneumonia (VAP) rates in surgical intensive care unit (SICU)	Provide safe, excellent quality of care for all patients	Reduce VAP in SICU	Achieve 30% reduction in SICU VAP from 4.6 to <2.0/1,000 device days	Use evidence-based practices to reduce VAP. Initiate Performance Improvement (PI) Team	Monitor monthly, report quarterly to staff and Infection Control Committee	Intensive care unit. Radiology technician. Medical staff. Invasive cardiac procedures. Other
Increased sharps injuries (scalpel) in the operating room (OR) staff	Provide safe work environment for employees	Reduce sharps injuries from scalpels	Reduce scalpel injuries to OR staff from 20 per quarter to less than 2 per quarter	PI Team. Review equipment; Review existing policy; update as necessary	Monitor monthly, report monthly to OR staff	Operating theater. Employee health. Surgeons. Infection control
Expected influx of patients with communicable disease during epidemic	Prepare organization for emergency situations	Develop and test plan for influx of infectious patients	Triage and care for up to 100 patients per day for 3 days with respiratory illness related to epidemic or pandemic	Develop triage and surge plan. Educate staff. Obtain supplies. Test plan and revise based on findings	Test three times by June 2007 with increasingly successful results in managing influx	Emergency room staff. Physicians. Administration. Admitting. Safety. Infection control. Other

Source: Barbara M. Soule. Used with permission.

beneficial interventions. First, it is essential to be aware of and use relevant evidence-based guidelines for practice. Many guidelines exist and are discussed throughout this book. The US CDC, WHO, Institute for Healthcare Improvement (IHI), and others have analyzed and synthesized research to make thoughtful recommendations, most of which can be found online (*see* the "Further Readings" section at the end of this chapter for Web links). For example, the IHI has identified the following bundles and components:

Central Line Bundle

- Hand hygiene
- Maximal barrier precautions on insertion
- Chlorhexidine skin antisepsis
- Optimal catheter site selection, with subclavian vein as the preferred site for nontunneled catheters
- Daily review of line necessity with prompt removal of unnecessary lines

Ventilator Bundle

- Elevation of the head of the bed
- Daily "sedation vacations" and assessment of readiness to extubate
- Peptic ulcer disease prophylaxis
- Deep venous thrombosis prophylaxis

Surgical Site Infection Bundle

- Appropriate use of antibiotics
- Appropriate hair removal
- Maintenance of postoperative glucose control for major cardiac surgical patients
- Postoperative normothermia for colorectal surgery patients[33]

Second is the use of surveillance data to guide action. For these data to be helpful, they must be accurate and complete. It is essential to use the surveillance data to make change. If data are collected and analyzed but not used to guide IPC activities, they are useless.[34] One of the key roles of the IPC practitioner is to translate data and information into practice improvement strategies and to function as an interventionist to initiate and guide improvement activities.[35] Principles of surveillance are discussed in the following section. A third tactic is to consider the various factors that contribute to successful change and integrate them into planning and execution. For example, including experienced, competent staff who are empowered to make changes in developing the strategies, and developing a culture that supports innovation and advocates for improvement are factors that may increase success. When an organization makes the

---

SIDEBAR 4-6

Characteristics of Successful Intervention Strategies

- Leadership support and commitment
- Culture fostering improvement and patient safety
- Multidisciplinary teams that include staff who understands the current process and can participate fully
- Practice leaders to serve as champions
- Performance improvement methods such as PDSA (Plan, Do, Study, Act) to help the change process and failure mode and effects analysis to address anticipated challenges (*see* Chapter 5)
- Policies and procedures that are clearly written and understood
- Education to share information and work toward competency
- Monitoring, auditing, and evaluating the change process at all stages
- Constant communication about the change for all appropriate persons and committees
- Creating permanence for successful changes (hardwiring into the culture)
- Celebrating success

Source: Adapted from Fauerbach L.L.: Infection control interventions: Key to prevention. In Arias K., Soule B. (eds.): *The APIC/JCAHO Infection Control Workbook.* Washington, D.C., and Oakbrook Terrace, IL: Association for Professionals in Infection Control and Epidemiology, Inc., and Joint Commission on Accreditation of Healthcare Organizations, 2006, pp. 67–84.

---

appropriate supplies available and provides time for implementation of new changes, these factors will also contribute to achieving the goal.

Intervention strategies may include such efforts as reducing a high rate of catheter-related bloodstream infections or infections after abdominal surgery, decreasing the incidence of VAP or UTIs, minimizing sharps injuries in health care workers, or preventing TB transmission in the acute or ambulatory care setting. Educating staff, making changes in policies and procedures, or reinforcing existing ones and providing feedback on current activities help improve performance. Often it is necessary to use all of these methods simultaneously. See Sidebar 4-6 above for a list of characteristics of successful intervention strategies.

Identifying Risks Through Surveillance, Data Collection, and Analysis

Surveillance is a fundamental aspect of an effective IPC program and an essential activity to determine high-risk areas that call for intervention strategies (PCI.11).[36–40]

Surveillance involves collecting data about infections and care practices for a variety of purposes, including the following:

- To assess an organization's risks for infection for patients, staff, and the environment
- To identify areas that need further investigation, such as areas where patients seem to be at higher risk
- To search out cases of a specific disease
- To identify cluster or outbreaks of infections and then intervene
- To determine whether processes used to prevent and control infections are effective and whether revisions or improvements to systems are necessary
- To determine education and policy needs
- To check the success of any changes made to a system or process
- To identify any problems such as the emergence of new infections or outbreaks such as severe acute respiratory syndrome (SARS) or influenza

Because infection risks change over time, data collection and risk assessment must be an ongoing process. Although constant monitoring is resource intensive, it is ultimately cost effective because many HAIs are preventable. The quantitative information an organization gets from data collection and measurement of activities can help reveal whether an IPC program is actually reducing the risk of infections and can demonstrate its value to leadership.

What to Collect

The surveillance data an organization collects and analyzes shows infection trends. This information forms the basis for IPC measures. Surveillance should be simple and practical. IPC professionals often have many duties and responsibilities. Scarce resources should be focused on the surveillance that will be most useful in improving patient safety and care outcomes. Although total surveillance may be ideal, it is not possible in many organizations. Focusing data collection efforts on infections that place patients at highest risk provides the most benefit from surveillance activities. For example, instead of tracking all UTIs, organizations might consider monitoring only those involving indwelling catheters in specific patient populations. Or the IPC program may focus only on central lines in the ICU.

There are two general types and many approaches to surveillance. The two general types of surveillance are described below followed by various methods.

The first type is process monitoring. Process monitors examine IPC processes or procedures *before and as* they are implemented (for example, monitoring could be focused on practices that are established in the organization to reduce infection risk). A process monitor could measure the frequency and consistency with which staff perform hand hygiene, how often physicians or nurses use appropriate barriers when inserting peripheral or central intravenous lines or an indwelling urinary catheter, or the timing of the administration of preoperative antibiotics prior to the surgical incision. The purpose of a process monitor is to determine whether policies and best practices that can minimize infection risk are being followed by staff. The second type of surveillance reviews outcomes. Outcome measures examine the results of IPC processes, patient care practices, or other procedures *after* they are implemented and performed. Outcome measures include the rates of UTIs, SSIs, and bloodstream infections. These rates indicate the quality of infection prevention and patient safety efforts. For health care workers, the number of staff who convert from TB negative skin test to TB positive is an outcome measure and may be compared with process measures related to appropriate isolation and TB medications for active pulmonary TB patients.

Many methods of surveillance can be used for either process or outcome surveillance.[36] Some of these measures are described below.

Focused Incidence Surveillance
Incidence surveillance looks at all new infections in a given time period (for example during one month or a year). Infections can be compared from one period to another when rates are calculated using denominators of persons at risk for the infection and those who actually get the infection. Incidence surveillance can be performed in a number of ways, including the following:

- Targeted surveillance—concentrates on specific patient populations or procedures. For example, in a primary health care organization, targeted surveillance might involve monitoring patients who receive enteral or parenteral feedings and who suffer a higher-than-expected incidence of diarrhea; or in an acute care setting, surveillance may be targeted to infections of patients in ICUs and patients with selected surgical procedures, or those at risk for bloodstream infections. Data from these targeted surveillance efforts will highlight areas that need improvement.
- Problem-oriented surveillance—performed to focus on identified infections that are problem areas and to measure the occurrence of these specific infections. When a cluster of patients have the same illness, surveillance efforts should involve an in-depth assessment to determine whether an ongoing problem exists and what control measures can be applied to address the problem.

Prevalence Surveillance
Prevalence surveillance monitors all infections (existing and new) during a given time period, such as one day, week, or month. For example, the IPC practitioner may want to look at the number of VAPs in a single ICU during a three-month period or the number of patients who come to an

ambulatory or primary health center with malaria in a week. One prevalence survey is like a photograph that captures only one point or period in time. A single prevalence survey is not always considered a reliable indicator for designing IPC interventions. However, repeated prevalence surveys of the same infection performed over time add validity to the data, increasing confidence. Prevalence surveillance is very intensive during the period being monitored but because the time period can be limited, this method provides opportunity for other IPC activities and is a cost-effective use of IPC practitioner resources.[41–44]

Although the types of data an organization collects during its surveillance efforts will depend on the organization's patient populations and services provided, the following list suggests some common organisms, areas, and groups to monitor or audit during surveillance efforts:

- Multiple drug-resistant organisms, such as methicillin-resistant *Staphylococcus aureus* (MRSA), vancomycin-resistant enterococci (VRE) (particularly in critical care areas), *Clostridium difficile* or others specific to the country or the organization
- Surgical-site infections
- Infections related to implanted devices
- Infections related to indwelling devices, such as urinary catheters and central intravenous lines
- Sharps or needlestick injuries in staff
- Emerging pathogens such as West Nile virus
- Hepatitis C infections in hemodialysis units
- Infections in immunocompromised patients
- Infections in patients with extremes of age (premature infants to frail elderly)

In choosing what data to collect, an organization should consider not only its patient population and services provided but also what data are available, accessible, and meaningful. Organizations can use their own staff as a resource to identify areas of concern and look both internally and externally for suggestions on common areas to monitor. Many of these areas will be identified in the risk assessment. The organization might choose to perform surveillance on process measures such as the use of isolation procedures, the cleaning of patient environments, appropriate barrier precautions during construction or renovation, or the use of appropriate procedures to prevent patients on ventilators from acquiring pneumonia. As described above, monitoring the rate of infections will provide the organization with outcome data. Employees can also provide valuable information on what activities put them and their patients at risk for infections. For example, are staff members having a large number of needlesticks, or acquiring HAIs during the course of their work? One process monitor might look at whether nurses and nurse aides are using proper precautions with residents with MRSA in a long term care facility.

How to Collect the Data

As there are several sources for IPC data, there are also several ways to collect it. Following are some practical suggestions on how to easily and thoroughly collect data for IPC efforts:

- Reporting systems. These systems allow staff to phone, e-mail, or write reports about patients with infections. When a cluster of infections is reported, IPC professionals, along with leadership, should take immediate action to address the infection and control its spread. Reporting systems are a passive approach to surveillance that relies on health care or laboratory personnel to report issues, so underreporting could be a problem. For organizations to overcome underreporting, they must make it easy for staff to report issues, avoid punishing staff members who report by blaming them for the issues, and respond to issues reported. Staff members must feel that by reporting they are helping to improve the safety of patients and helping to decrease infections across the organization. Providing feedback for staff members who report potential infections will help establish value and strengthen their commitment to this process.
- Record review. There are a variety of records from which organizations can collect data regarding infections, including the following:
  - Admission logs
  - Employee health records
  - Incident reports
  - Laboratory records
  - Patient records
  - Pharmacy records
  - Reports on numbers/types of diagnostic workups and care recipient disposition
  - Treatment plans

  Organizations can review records for surveillance data through automated means or manually. These capabilities will depend on the size and scope of the organization's activities and the resources available. Computers and software significantly ease the data collection process. Although data can be collected manually, electronic programs can sort and analyze data and generate rates, graphs, charts, and reports.
- Walking rounds. This data collection method allows IPC staff to collect infection data on weekly or daily rounds, depending on the organization's size. During rounds, IPC staff consult with other staff and make clinical observations. During this time, IPC staff can also review charts, laboratory or radiology reports, treatment plans, and antibiotic or culture reports.

- Forms. Many organizations create simple tools to collect data regarding surveillance measures. For example, an organization can create a form on which staff members note their use of antibiotics. Information from this form can be converted into a chart or graph that when taken in aggregate will quickly reveal antibiotic use trends over time. Pharmacists can generate similar data.
- Data mining. This is an evolving process that is becoming important with the advancement of information technology systems. Data mining identifies important patterns, associations, changes, anomalies, and structures from a variety of sources, such as patient records or incident reports[45], through the use of a specialized computer program that might reveal trends not shown by traditional record review methods.
- Literature reviews. Although internal data are important in the discovery of infections, IPC professionals should also review the IPC literature and information from IPC organizations and governmental agencies for important HAIs that are occurring and emerging in other organizations. Reliable sources for this type of information include the following:
  - The World Health Organization (WHO)
  - The U.S. Centers for Disease Control and Prevention (US CDC) and the Division of Healthcare Quality and Promotion (DHQP)
  - National Safety and Healthcare Network (NSHN)
  - The Association for Professionals in Infection Control and Epidemiology (APIC)
  - *American Journal of Infection Control and Epidemiology*
  - Society for Healthcare Epidemiology of America (SHEA)
  - *Infection Control and Hospital Epidemiology* (journal)
  - International Federation of Infection Control (IFIC)
  - *Journal of Hospital Infection*
  - IPC journals from other countries

  Other resources can be found in Appendix 3 and at the end of each chapter.

From this research, IPC professionals can determine whether their organization should be collecting internal data on these new infections and what, if any, control measures need to be put in place.

Benchmarking

Although it is important to collect data, it is even more important to do something with the data after they are collected. Data without analysis are just data. One of the most effective ways to analyze the data is through benchmarking. The benchmarking process compares the organization's data with a reliable, scientifically based set of data that the organization believes represents desired or best practice. Benchmarking, with data feedback to clinicians and quality management professionals, accounts for the most significant and enduring changes for improvement in managing infections.[46,47]

Organizations can benchmark against themselves and also with external sources such as the WHO's *Weekly Epidemiological Record* or the US CDC's National Safety Health Network (NHSN) (formerly, the Nosocomial Infections Surveillance [NNIS]) reports. Internal sources help illustrate success in improving performance over time, whereas external benchmarking can help reveal higher-than-average rates of complications that can highlight larger issues.

Internal Benchmarking

The first step in effectively benchmarking data is to establish performance rates. This begins with generating a baseline to get an initial picture of the organization and to which subsequent data can be compared. Looking at absolute numbers of infections is misleading. By calculating rates and comparing data over time periods to the initial baseline, an organization can see whether the infection rate is increasing or decreasing. Rates are critical in tracking performance, trending variance, measuring statistical significance, and calculating an acceptable target rate. If multiple departments are determining infection rates that are comparable, it can be a useful exercise to benchmark data within departments or units.

External Benchmarking

This is the comparison of organization data with external sources over time. Although there are many choices of benchmark data to use, the following are some suggestions:
- Similar settings across a specific geographic area
- Medical practices literature or other professional, recognized standards of practice
- Databases, including the following:
  - WHO's *Weekly Epidemiological Record*
  - National Health Safety Network database at the US CDC. The NHSN has been aggregating surveillance data from participating hospitals since 1970 using standardized protocols for adult and pediatric ICUs, high-risk nurseries, and surgical patients. Infections are categorized using standard definitions from the US CDC.

To successfully benchmark data, whether internally or externally, an organization needs to use measures that have standardized and uniform definitions and methods for data collection and risk adjustment. This allows the organization to compare apples to apples and get an accurate picture of how well its IPC program is doing. It is also important to benchmark against the highest standards so that the organization continues to strive to meet and exceed the best benchmarks.

In some cases, such as within certain behavioral health care organizations, comparisons with the rates of other similar organizations might not be effective because of case-mix variation. In this situation, comparing rates internally over time within the organization has more impact on evaluating what is really happening.

Whenever an organization revises a process or creates a new one, it should determine how its effectiveness can be measured. It is important to use process surveillance indicators directly applicable to the new or revised practice. Examples of this type of thinking appear in the IPC guidelines available from or under development at the WHO and US CDC. In its 2003 recommendations on preventing infections in the health care environment, the US CDC included five performance measures to help evaluate the usefulness of those recommendations.[48] Also, the draft of updated patient isolation guidelines, currently under review, includes administrative, process, outcome, and surveillance measures to use as quality indicators. Organizations might want to review these and similar guidelines for examples of how to determine what types of information should be used to measure their own processes.

Reporting Data to External Agencies

In addition to collecting data for internal improvement processes, it is important to gather information to aid in the early identification of infection clusters, outbreaks, bioterrorist threats, or new diseases. Public health or national agencies in some countries perform their own monitoring activities to help with early identification. They also rely on organizations to rapidly report unusual trends and patterns. If an organization does not have an effective system in place for reporting to public health organizations, then the likelihood of rapid disease and outbreak identification is diminished. To make sure that trends and patterns are reported to the appropriate authorities, organizations should have policies and procedures that comply with local reporting laws. The Ministry of Health in Saudi Arabia requires all hospitals to report within 24 hours all cases of meningococcal meningitis. These reports are received by the 24-hour on-call Ministry of Health staff who promptly initiate contact tracing and preventive vaccination to all possible contacts.

Evaluating the Infection Prevention and Control Program: Goals, Objectives, and Strategies

Periodically (at least annually), the goals, objectives, strategies, and results should be evaluated by the IPC team and the IC committee to make sure that prevention methods are working and that infections and infection risks are being reduced to the minimum. The evaluation process identifies which activities have been successful and which should be changed to achieve better results.

Figure 4-3

Annual Evaluation Process

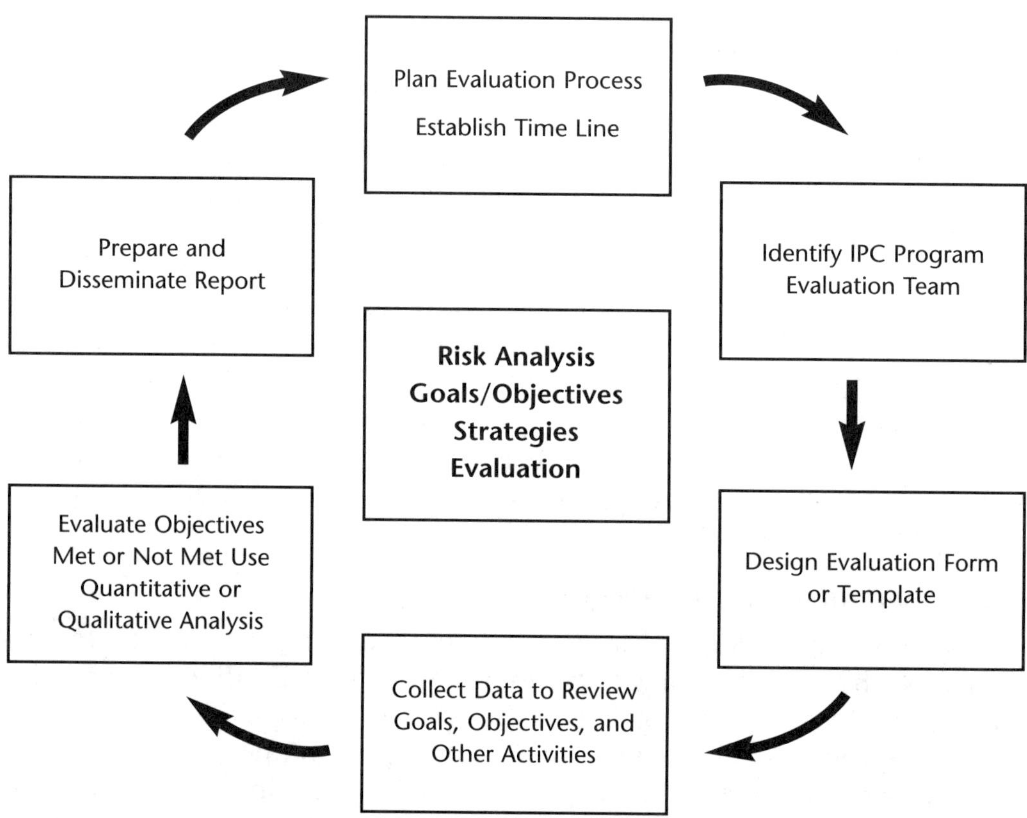

Source: Barbara M. Soule, R.N., M.P.A., C.I.C. Used with permission. This figure first appeared in Arias K., Soule B. (eds.): *The APIC/JCAHO Infection Control Workbook.* Washington, D.C., and Oakbrook Terrace, IL: Association for Professionals in Infection Control and Epidemiology, Inc., and Joint Commission on Accreditation of Healthcare Organizations, 2006, p. 86.

The evaluation should be performed as a multidisciplinary effort in a systematic and purposeful way. The IC committee should determine the evaluation time line and method to be used and how the results will be disseminated and integrated into the next risk and planning cycle prior to beginning the evaluation process. To perform the evaluation, the team will have to collate the results and data related to each of the objectives and strategies. In addition to the formal objectives, the evaluation should include an analysis of any clusters or outbreaks, significant policy changes, unusual deaths, and other pertinent events. Using this collective information, the team can perform the evaluation, record the findings, prepare a report, and disseminate the information to the staff and leadership of the organization. As with the risk assessment, numbers or terms or both can be used to evaluate the program (*see* Figure 4-3 above).

Conclusion

By creating an IPC program that continuously assesses risks for the acquisition and transmission of infectious agents, an organization can develop a planned approach to address and minimize or eliminate risks and evaluate how these approaches affect infection outcomes. When the program is in place, the organization must be continually vigilant for new and ongoing issues that must be assessed and addressed to prevent HAIs. Maintaining focus on IPC is often a challenge, and Chapter 5, "Maintaining an Effective Infection Prevention and Control Program: More Challenges, Tips, and Tools," provides strategies to meet this test.

References

1. Joint Commission Resources: JCAHO strengthening its infection standards. *Joint Commission Benchmark,*11:19–20, Feb. 2004

2. Ward M.M., et al.: Implementation of strategies to prevent and control the emergence and spread of antimicrobial-resistant microorganisms in U.S. hospitals. *Infect Control Hosp Epidemiol* 26:21–30, Jan. 2005.

3. Shuttleworth A.: The role of modern matrons in raising standards of infection control. *Nurs Times* 100:61, 63, Jun. 29–Jul. 6, 2004.

4. Shewchuk M.: Leaders' role in infection prevention and control: Fighting the invisible and invincible . . . if only . . . *Can Oper Room Nurs J.* 22:18, 21–22, 36, Jun. 2004.

5. Sriratanaban J., Wanavanichkul Y.: Hospitalwide quality improvement in Thailand. *Jt Comm J Qual Saf.* 30:246–256, May 2004.

6. Antoniak J.: Handwashing compliance. *Can Nurse* 100:21–25, Sep. 2004.

7. Zejda J.E.: [Professional profiles of physicians certified in epidemiology in the view of hospital managers in the Silesian Voivodeship of Poland]: *Przegl Epidemiol* 57(1):1–8, 2003.

8. Dembry L.M., Hierholzer W.J. Jr.: Educational needs and opportunities for the hospital epidemiologist. *Infect Control Hosp Epidemiol* 17:188–192, Mar. 1996.

9. Mylotte J.M.: The hospital epidemiologist in long-term care: Practical considerations. *Infect Control Hosp Epidemiol* 2:439–442, Jul. 1991.

10. Haley R.W.: The "hospital epidemiologist" in U.S. hospitals, 1976–1977: A description of the head of the infection surveillance and control program: Report from the SENIC project. *Infect Control* 1:21–32, Jan.–Feb. 1980.

11. Warren D.K., Kollef M.H.: Prevention of hospital infection. *Microbes Infect* 7:268–274, Feb. 2005.

12. Scheckler W.E., et al.: Requirements for infrastructure and essential activities of infection control and epidemiology in hospitals: A consensus panel report. Society for Healthcare Epidemiology of America. *Infect Control Hosp Epidemiol* 19:114–124, Feb. 1998.

13. Moro M.L., et al.: Infection control programs in Italian hospitals. *Infect Control Hosp Epidemiol* 25:36–40, Jan. 2004.

14. Pearse J.: Infection control in Africa: Nosocomial infection. *Afr Health* 19:10–11, Sep. 1997.

15. Murphy C.L., McLaws M.L.: Variation in administrators' and clinicians' attitudes toward critical elements of an infection control program and the role of the infection control practitioner in New South Wales, Australia. *Am J Infect Control* 29:262–270, Aug. 2001.

16. Burke J.P.: Infection control—A problem for patient safety. *N Engl J Med* 348:651–656, Feb. 13, 2003.

17. Gerberding J.L.: Hospital-onset infections: A patient safety issue. *Ann Intern Med* 137:665–670, Oct. 15, 2002.

18. O'Boyle C., Jackson M., Henly S.J.: Staffing requirements for infection control programs in US health care facilities: Delphi project. *Am J Infect Control* 30:321–333, Oct. 2002.

19. Ross K.A.: A program for infection surveillance utilizing an infection control liaison nurse. *Am J Infect Control* 10:24–28, Feb. 1982.

20. Ching T.Y., Seto W.H.: Evaluating the efficacy of the infection control liaison nurse in the hospital. *J Adv Nurs* 15:1128–1131, Oct. 1990.

21. Roberts C., Casey D.: An infection control link nurse network in the care home setting. *Br J Nurs* 13:166–170, Feb. 12–25, 2004.

22. Dawson S.J.: The role of the infection control link nurse. *J Hosp Infect* 54:251–257; quiz 320, Aug. 2003.

23. Teare E.L., Peacock A.: The development of an infection control link-nurse programme in a district general hospital. *J Hosp Infect* 34:267–278, Dec. 1996.

24. Pirwitz S.: The Certification Board of Infection Control, Inc. *Infect Control Hosp Epidemiol* 16:518–521, Sep. 1995.

25. Cookson B., Drasar B.: Diploma in hospital infection control—Important changes to the accreditation of prior experiential learning and update. *J Hosp Infect* 62:507–510, Apr. 2006.

26. Goldrick B.A., et al.: Practice analysis for infection control and epidemiology in the new millennium. *Am J Infect Control* 30:437–448, Dec. 2002.

27. Geubbels E.L.., et al.: Reduced risk of surgical site infections through surveillance in a network. *Int J Qual Health Care* 18:127–133, Apr. 2006.

28. Construction-related nosocomial infections in patients in health care facilities: Decreasing the risk of *Aspergillus, Legionella* and other infections. *Can Commun Dis Rep* 27 (suppl. 2):i–x, 1–42, i–x, 1–46, Jul. 2001.

29. Weinberg M., et al.: Reducing infections among women undergoing cesarean section in Colombia by means of continuous quality improvement methods. *Arch Intern Med* 161:2357–2365, Oct. 22, 2001.

30. Larson E., Aiello A.E.: Systematic risk assessment methods for the infection control professional. *Am J Infect Control* 34:323–326, Jun. 2006.

31. Health and Safety Commission: *Five Steps to Risk Assessment.* http://www.hse.gov.uk/workplacetransport/information/riskassessment.htm (accessed Jul. 13, 2006).

32. O'Boyle C.: Qualitative analysis. In Carrick, R (ed.): *APIC Text of Infection Control and Epidemiology,* 2nd ed. Washington, D.C.: Association for Professionals in Infection Control and Epidemiology, Inc., 2005, pp. 30-1–30-9.

33. Institute for Healthcare Improvement: *Bundle Up for Safety.* http://www.ihi.org/IHI/Topics/CriticalCare/IntensiveCare/ImprovementStories/BundleUpforSafety.htm (accessed Jul. 26, 2006).

34. Lowett L.L., Massanari R.M.: Role of surveillance in emerging health sytems: Measurement is essential but not sufficient. *Am J Infect Control* 27:134–140, Apr. 1999.

35. Murphy D.M.: From expert data collectors to interventionists: Changing the focus for infection control professionals. *Am J Infect Control* 30:120–132, Apr. 2002.

36. Arias K.: Surveillance. In Carrick R. (ed.): *APIC Text of Infection Control and Epidemiology,* 2nd ed. Washington, D.C.: Association for Professionals in Infection Control and Epidemiology, Inc., 2005.

37. Lee T.B. et al.: Recommended practices for surveillance. Association for Professionals in Infection Control and Epidemiology, Inc. Surveillance Initiative Working Group. *Am J Infect Control* 26:277–288, Jun. 1998.

38. Pottinger J.M., Herwaldt L.A., Peri T.M.: Basics of surveillance—An overview. *Infect Control Hosp Epidemiol* 18:513–527, Jul. 1997.

39. Haley R.W.: The scientific basis for using surveillance and risk factor data to reduce nosocomial infection rates. *J Hosp Infect* 30 (suppl.):3–14, Jun. 2005.

40. French G., Friedman C. (eds.): *Infection Control: Basic Concepts and Practices.* 2nd ed. International Federation of Infection Control. 2003. http://www.theific.org/oldsite/Manual/toc.htm (accessed Jul. 10, 2006).

41. Balkhy H.H., et al.: Hospital- and community-acquired infections: A point prevalence and risk factors survey in a tertiary care center in Saudi Arabia. *Int J Infect Dis* 10:326–333, Jul. 2006.

42. Klavs I., et al.; Slovenian Hospital-Acquired Infections Survey Group: Prevalance of and risk factors for hospital-acquired infections in Slovenia— Results of the first national survey, 2001. *J Hosp Infect* 54:149–157. Jun. 2003.

43. Gikas A. et al.; Greek Infection Control Network: Prevalence study of hospital-acquired infections in 14 Greek hospitals: Planning from the local to the national surveillance level. *J Hosp Infect* 50:269–275, Apr. 2002.

44. Sodano L. et al.: [The prevalence survey of nosocomial infections: A very informative tool in a big hospital setting] [Article in Italian]. *Ann Ig* 16:647–663, Sep.–Oct. 2004.

45. Peterson L.: First alerts: Data vs. people methods of surveillance. Paper presented at the Joint Commission on Accreditation of Healthcare Organization's Infection Control Conference, Chicago, Nov. 17, 2003.

46. Richards C., et al.: Promoting quality through measurement of performance and response: Prevention success stories. *Emerg Infect Dis* 7:299–301, Mar.–Apr. 2001.

47. Gaynes R., et al., and the NNIS System Hospitals for the CDC: Feeding back surveillance data to prevent hospital-acquired infections. *Emerg Infect Dis* 7:295–298, Mar.–Apr. 2001.

48. Sehulster L., Chinn R.Y.W.: Guidelines for *Environmental Infection Control in Health-Care Facilities.* Washington, D.C.: National Center for Infectious Diseases, 2003.

Further Readings

Healthcare Infection Control Practices Advisory Committee (HICPAC): [Selected Guidelines: Guidance and Recommendations from the Centers for Disease Control and Prevention (CDC)]. http://www.cdc.gov/ncidod/dhqp/ hicpac_pubs.html.

Institute for Healthcare Improvement: *Surgical Site Infections: How to Improve.* http://www.ihi.org/IHI/Topics/PatientSafety/SurgicalSiteInfections/ HowToImprove/.

World Health Organization (WHO), Regional Office for South-East Asia and Regional Office for Western Pacific: *Practical Guidelines for Infection Control in Health Care Facilities.* WHO. 2004. http://www.wpro.who.int/NR/rdonlyres/006EF250-6B11-42B4-BA17-C98D413BE8B8/0/practical_guidelines_infection_control.pdf.

Resources

The following readings were gathered for use in *Information Resources in Infection Control,* Fourth Edition (Editor: Nizam Damani M.D., MBBS, MSc, FRCPI, FRCPath), due in 2006 from the International Federation of Infection Control (IFIC). The full document will be available online at IFIC's Web site: http://www.theific.org/publications.asp. NOTE: Some of these resources may appear at the end of more than one chapter, due to their applicability to more than one aspect of infection prevention and control.

American Thoracic Society and the Infectious Diseases Society of America: Guidelines for the management of adults with hospital-acquired, ventilator-associated, and healthcare-associated pneumonia. *Am J Respir CritCare Med* 171:388–416, Feb. 2005.

Association for Professionals in Infection Control and Epidemiology, Inc.: APIC Surveillance Initiative Working Group. Recommended practice for surveillance. *Am J Infect Control* 26:277–288, Jun. 1998.

Centers for Disease Control and Prevention: Guidelines for Prevention of Nosocomial Pneumonia. *MMWR Morb Mortal Wkly Rep* 46(RR-1):1–79, 1997. http://www.cdc.gov/mmwr/preview/mmwrhtml/00045365.htm.

————: CDC definitions of surgical sites infections, 1992: A modification of the CDC definitions of wound infections. *Am J Infect Control* 20:271–274, Oct. 1992.

Cruse P.J.E., Foord R.: The epidemiology of wound infections: A 10-year prospective study of 62,939 wounds. *Surg Clin North Am* 60:27–40, Feb. 1980.

————: A five-year prospective study of 23,649 surgical wounds. *Arch Surg* 107:206–210, Aug. 1973.

Department of Health (UK): Guidelines for preventing infections associated with the insertion and maintenance central venous catheters. *J Hosp Infect* 47 (suppl.):S47–S67, 2001. http://www.dh.gov.uk/assetRoot/04/07/73/68/04077368.PDF.

Department of Health (UK): Guidelines for preventing infections associated with the insertion and maintenance of short-term indwelling urethral catheters in acute care. *J Hosp Infect* 47 (suppl.):S39–S46, Oct. 2001.

Emmerson A.M., et al.: The Second National Prevalence Survey of Infection in Hospitals—Overview of the results. *J Hosp Infect* 32:175–190, Jan. 1996.

Gaynes R.P., et al.: Surgical site infection (SSI) rates in the United States, 1992–1998: The NNIS basic risk index. *Clin Infect Dis* 33 (suppl. 2):S69–S77, Sep. 2001.

Glenister H.M., et al.: *A Study of Surveillance Methods for Detecting Hospital Infection*. London: Public Health Laboratory Service, 1992.

Glynn A., et al.: *Hospital-Acquired Infection: Surveillance, Policies and Practice*. London: Public Health Laboratory Service, 1997.

Haley R.W., et al.: The efficacy of infection surveillance and control programs in preventing nosocomial infection in US hospitals. (SENIC study). *Am J Epidemiol* 121(2):182–205.

Health Protection Agency: *Protocol for Surveillance of Surgical Site Infection*. 2004. www.hpa.org.uk/.

Hospital Infection Society (UK): Behaviours and rituals in the operating theatre. *J Hosp Infect* 51:241–255, Aug. 2002. http://www.his.org.uk/_db/_documents/OTIC-final.pdf.

Infection Control Nurses Association (IFNA): *Guidelines for Preventing Intravascular Catheter-Related Infection*. Bathgate, UK: IFNA, 2001.

Klaucke D.N. et al.: Guidelines for evaluating surveillance systems. *MMWR Morb Mortal Wkly Rep* 37 (suppl. 5):1–18, May 6, 1988. http://www.cdc.gov/mmwr/preview/mmwrhtml/00001769.htm.

Mangram A. et al.: CDC guideline for prevention of surgical site infection. *Infect Control Hosp Epidemiol* 20(4):247–280, 1999.

McGeer A., et al.: Definitions of infection for surveillance in long term care facilities. *Am J Infect Control* 19(1):1–7, 1991.

Mermel L.A., et al.: Guidelines for the management of intravascular catheter-related infections. *Clin Infect Dis* 32(9):1249–1272, 2001.

Nicolle L.E.: Urinary tract infections in long-term-care facilities (SHEA Position Paper). *Infect Control Hosp Epidemiol* 22:167–175, Sep. 2001.

O'Grady N.P., et al.; Healthcare Infection Control Practices Advisory Committee. Guidelines for the prevention of intravascular catheter-related infections. *Infect Control Hosp Epidemiol* 23:759–769, 2002. http://www.shea-online.org/Assets/files/position_papers/hicpac_catheter.pdf.

Public Health Agency of Canada: Preventing infections associated with indwelling intravascular access devices. *Can Commun Dis Rep* 23S8, Dec. 1997.

Public Health Laboratory Service (PHLS): *Socioeconomic Burden of Hospital-Acquired Infection*. London: PHLS, 1999.

Tablan O.C., et al., Centers for Disease Control and Prevention: Guidelines for preventing healthcare associated pneumonia, 2003. *MMWR Morb Mortal Wkly Rep* 53(RR-03):1–36, 2004. http://www.cdc.gov/mmwr/preview/mmwrhtml/rr5303a1.htm.

CHAPTER FIVE

Maintaining an Effective Infection Prevention and Control Program

More Challenges, Tips, and Tools

When an infection prevention and control (IPC) program is in place with appropriate leadership support, goals and objectives, staff, policies and procedures, surveillance and intervention strategies, and effective communication and education mechanisms, organizations must continue to assess risks, maintain or implement specific interventions to address the risks, and evaluate the results.

One aspect of this ongoing vigilance is to recognize that unanticipated deaths, even when associated with infection, are adverse events and should be managed as such. This means that they should undergo a root cause analysis to understand why the patient acquired an infection and why, after the infection had occurred, the patient died. It is important to learn not only why infections occur but how to treat patients successfully when they do acquire infections. For more information about deaths and injuries related to health care–associated infections, please see the *Sentinel Event Alert* on this topic from the Joint Commission on Accreditation of Healthcare Organizations. It is available at no cost online at http://www.jointcommission.org/SentinelEvents/SentinelEventAlert/sea_28.htm.

Responding to Identified Risks and Performance Deficits: An Ongoing Process

During IPC activities such as surveillance for infections, environmental rounds, observations of care delivery practices, and discussions with health care workers, IPC staff should pay close attention to outcomes and undesirable trends and examine the processes associated with the identified high-risk areas. Following are some questions organizations should ask to make sure that IPC policies and procedures are appropriate and that actual practice reflects the stated requirements:[1]

- What systems/processes/policies currently put patients, staff, and others at risk for infections? Which systems have been effective in minimizing infections?
- Are the appropriate systems/processes/policies in place to help prevent infections?
- Have staff been oriented to policies and procedures, surveillance data, and reporting processes and procedures?
- Are staff following organizational IPC policies?
- Is information about infections reported internally (for performance improvement) and externally to public health agencies?

Based on the responses to these and other questions, organizations can evaluate system breakdowns or performance deficits and develop specific interventions to improve practice. This might involve creating a new program or education initiative, implementing a performance improvement team, or updating, revising, and creating new policies as necessary. System issues can also be addressed using performance improvement tools and multidisciplinary teams (*see* Chapter 4). For example, if surveillance identifies an increase in catheter-related bloodstream infections and additional, focused surveillance indicates that the appropriate sterile barriers are not being used during the insertion of central intravenous lines, this may indicate the lack of a clear policy and procedure, lack of staff knowledge or understanding of the policy, inadequate compliance with the stated requirements for the insertion of central lines into the bloodstream, or unavailable or inappropriate equipment for the procedure. Each of these factors should be considered when performance variation is identified and analyzed (*see* Sidebar 5-1 on page 113).

In a continual process of improvement, and depending on the scope of the initiative, an organization might want to apply a quality improvement (QI) methodology such as Plan-Do-Study-Act (PDSA), Six Sigma, or failure mode and effects analysis (FMEA) to use surveillance information to guide the initiative improvement process. PDSA is a four-step method for delineating quality issues, planning, implementing, testing and integrating methods to improve the quality of processes.[2] Six Sigma is a data-driven improvement methodology that strives for near perfection in eliminating defects (driving toward six standard deviations between the mean and the nearest specification limit) in any process.[3] FMEA is a systematic assessment that examines a process in detail before it is implemented. The evaluation includes the sequencing of events and actual and potential risks, failures, or points of vulnerability and the impact on clients (criticality). Areas for

SIDEBAR 5-1

Analyzing Reasons for Performance Discrepancies

An important function of every infection prevention and control (IPC) program is to understand the nature of performance discrepancies. When personnel do not follow approved practices, the result is a performance discrepancy that may increase infection risk and need to be corrected or improved. The infection control committee or IPC staff may be responsible for recommending the corrective action. If the nature of the performance discrepancy is correctly identified, and the system issues addressed, improvement is likely to follow.

Below are three common reasons for performance deficits:

- **Lack of knowledge** (personnel do not know how to perform the task correctly, or they do not understand the policy or process or why it is important).
- **Inadequate system support,** such as lack of equipment or barriers to getting or using the equipment (personnel know how to do the task, but the equipment does not support the task or is unavailable or does not work) or other barriers in the system preventing the desired behavior.
- **Lack of motivation or management reinforcement** to perform the task correctly (personnel know how, and the equipment is appropriate, but they still do the task incorrectly).

Developing skills to evaluate which of these reasons contribute to an inadequate performance, along with looking at each as part of a system, will increase the likelihood that corrective action will be successful. For example, fiber-optic endoscopes are challenging to clean and disinfect, and the use of an improperly cleaned endoscope could result in health care–associated infections. Providing instruction for personnel on how to do the job better will improve the situation only if the cleaning and disinfecting equipment is adequate, and the cleaning personnel are given the time and incentive to perform the job correctly. If an automated endoscope washer fails to clean properly, an education program for staff members will not improve the situation. Likewise, if personnel rush through the job because there are too few endoscopes for the number of procedures, education and new cleaning brushes will not improve the situation. Hand hygiene is another example. If staff members know how to clean their hands and know when it is appropriate to do so, and if alcohol-based hand rub or soap and water and towels are available but personnel still do not wash their hands properly, they may not fully understand the importance of hand hygiene, they may lack incentive, or they may be "too busy." There might also be an absence of management insistence that hand hygiene is expected for all employees. Lack of hand hygiene may go unnoticed, and compliance with the hand hygiene policy may be unrewarded.

When the issue is identified and addressed, the organization should ensure that the desired performance is acknowledged and rewarded and that inadequate performance is corrected. Purposefully addressing performance issues using this simple framework with a focus on how the system supports or inhibits performance may help improve processes and outcomes and reduce infection risks for patients and staff.

Further Reading

Mager R.F., Pipe, P.: *Analyzing Performance Problems.* Atlanta: Center for Effective Performance, 1997.

improvement are prioritized based on this process.[4] Any of these methods, if used correctly and with leadership support, are likely to improve practice.

As with the development of the IPC program, specific interventions to improve patient care and reduce infection risk should involve key players in the organization. It is helpful to have a multidisciplinary team design, implement, and monitor specific interventions regarding IPC. For example, when creating an organizationwide hand hygiene program, representatives from nursing, medical staff, environment of care, housekeeping, food service, and administration can all provide valuable input and support.

After an initiative is designed and implemented, staff should periodically measure the results to determine whether the initiative is meeting its objectives, the desired results are sustained, and new or revised IPC needs are identified. An organization might want to use incidence data or a "point prevalence" or "period prevalence" study to periodically audit or monitor the success of a particular initiative. As described in Chapter 4, incidence data monitor *new* events during a given time period. For example, if the improvement objective is to increase the use of appropriate sterile barriers during insertion of central lines, incidence data would look at each *new* instance when these barriers were not used during the surveillance period. Incidence or ongoing surveillance is a valuable way to evaluate effectiveness. It can also be resource intensive. An alternative is using the prevalence method. Prevalence surveillance identifies all instances of inadequate barriers during a defined period of time (day, month). The findings from each measurement period are compared with the previous results. Consistent findings provide confidence that the situation is stable. If there are significant changes, further analyses are performed to understand why the rates have increased or decreased. Point and period prevalence surveillance is an efficient and cost-effective way to achieve ongoing performance monitoring.[5]

Specific Interventions to Reduce the Spread of Infection

Depending on the organization, different interventions will focus on IPC. The following section discusses some IPC interventions and offers tips and strategies for implementation.

Hand Hygiene

The hands of health care workers are a major source of infectious agents.[6,7] Microorganisms can be transmitted from such obviously contaminated sources as purulent sputum or drainage from an infected wound, but can also be spread through contact with less obvious sources such as normal intact human skin, items in the patient environment (for example, over-bed tables, urinals, bedpans), and devices used in the care setting (for example, computer keyboards and telephones, which are also often colonized or contaminated with potentially pathogenic microorganisms[8–10]). These latter sources may not be visibly soiled and, therefore, not viewed as reservoirs of organisms, but in some cases they have been implicated in disease transmission. Some "clean" activities, such as taking a pulse or blood pressure or lifting a patient, may result in acquiring significant transient organisms that can be transmitted to others.

Hand hygiene is one of the most effective ways to prevent the spread of infection. Donald Berwick, president and CEO of the Institute for Healthcare Improvement (IHI), estimates that hospitals could save upward of 100,000 lives per year if they imposed a zero tolerance policy for workers failing to perform hand hygiene when indicated. In fact, IHI's 100,000 Lives Campaign did save an estimated 122,300 lives during an 18-month period in 2005–2006.[11] There are also economic arguments in support of improved hand hygiene. Some are cited by the World Health Organization (WHO) in the *WHO Guidelines on Hand Hygiene in Health Care* (Advanced Draft), published in 2005. Among those discussed by the WHO are the following:

- The excess use of hospital resources associated with only four or five health care–associated infections of average severity may equal the entire annual budget for hand hygiene products used in inpatient care areas.
- A single severe infection of a surgical site, lower respiratory tract, or bloodstream may cost the hospital more than its entire annual budget for antiseptic agents used for hand hygiene.
- In a neonatal intensive care unit (ICU) in the Russian Federation, the excess cost of one health care–associated bloodstream infection (US$1,100) would cover 3,265 patient-days of hand antiseptic use (US$0.34 per patient-day).
- The alcohol-based hand rub applied for hand hygiene in this unit would be cost-effective if its use prevented only 8.5 pneumonias or 3.5 bloodstream infections each year.[7]

Hand hygiene is a major factor in breaking the chain of infection in an effective IPC program. Hand hygiene is a simple act, and yet many health care organizations have significant trouble achieving acceptable staff compliance rates. Some researchers have measured mean baseline rates of 5% to 81% and an overall average of 40%.[12] Although health care workers do not generally or intentionally avoid washing their hands, they may be "too busy" or too distracted or may not value the importance of rigorous hand hygiene enough to engage in the activity as well as they should. Hand hygiene is a requirement of Joint Commission International's (JCI's) International Patient Safety Goals. Organizations should implement WHO or U.S. Centers for Disease Control and Prevention (US CDC) guidelines— or another evidence-based set of guidelines that is published and generally accepted—to ensure proper hand hygiene within the organization (*see* Chapters 1 and 2 for more information on this topic).

How do organizations improve the hand hygiene practices of their staff and work toward proper hand hygiene organizationwide? The case study on pages 119–120 provides guidance, and other suggestions are listed below.

Educate Staff

In some cases, health care workers are not aware of the activities that cause hand contamination. Dressing an open wound is a procedure in which it is likely that most staff would wash their hands (in addition to wearing gloves). Less obvious procedures such as touching the patient's immediate care environment might not be viewed as requiring hand hygiene. In addition, because there is a delay between improper hand hygiene and the emergence of an infection, many health care providers do not see the cause-and-effect relationship between thoroughly cleaning their hands and preventing infection. For staff to realize the importance of proper hand hygiene and engage in it at appropriate times, organizations should provide information on when hand hygiene is appropriate, as well as data and research that illustrate the importance of hand hygiene and feedback about their performance. This information can be incorporated into staff in-services, on posters displayed in patient and staff break rooms, or through organization newsletters and bulletins. Multiple educational approaches should be used simultaneously to maximize behavior change.[12] IPC practitioners should consider and incorporate the different learning preferences of staff into their teaching methods (*see* Table 5-1 on page 117).

Even if staff see value in hand hygiene, there might be some confusion as to when it is appropriate to use hand rubs versus hand washing. Organizations should educate staff members about the appropriate times to wash their hands versus using an alcohol-based hand rub. For example, when hands are visibly dirty or contaminated with proteinaceous material or are visibly soiled with blood or other body fluids, or after using the toilet, staff should wash their hands with soap and water. If hands are not visibly soiled, staff can use soap and water or an alcohol-based hand rub for routinely decontaminating hands. For certain organisms that exist in spore forms (for example, *Clostridium difficile*), hand washing is recommended to mechanically remove the spores.[6,7]

Create a Culture That Promotes Hygiene

For staff to regularly comply with hand hygiene procedures, an organization should foster a culture of safety—an expectation or an atmosphere in which errors never or seldom occur because staff are trained to avoid practices and circumstances that produce errors. In such a culture of safety, hand hygiene is expected, and it is unacceptable not to perform hand hygiene according to policy. Some have used the term "zero tolerance" to promote an organizational culture to prevent infections.[13] This type of culture already exists in certain areas of health care. For example, in the

TABLE 5-1

Learning Preferences Based on Multiple Intelligences

Learning Preference	Teaching Method
Verbal/Linguistic	Language, Words, Readings
Logical/Mathematics	Numbers, Puzzles, Problems
Visual/Spatial	Images, Pictures, Photos, Videos
Bodily/Kinesthetic	Practice, Return Demonstrations
Musical/Sound	Auditory, Lectures, Stories
Interpersonal	People, Teamwork, Collaborative Projects
Introspective	Reflection, Analysis

Source: Adapted from Gardner, H.: *Multiple Intelligences: The Theory in Practice.* New York: Basic Books, 1993.

operating theater, surgeons do not perform surgery and staff do not assist without having performed a preoperative scrub.

This culture of safety is often absent in other settings, and staff may be quite reluctant to challenge those with more authority to comply with hygienic protocols. To achieve full hand hygiene compliance, a culture of expectation must be reinforced by leadership. Studies have shown that when administration makes overt and strong statements that hand hygiene is important, behavior is more likely to change.[14,15]

Organizations cannot expect overnight transformation, however, because behavioral changes are difficult to initiate and slow to become part of the workplace culture. To track changes in culture and identify areas for continued work, it is important to periodically monitor hand hygiene adherence with observational studies and provide feedback to personnel about their performance.[6]

Make Hand Hygiene Convenient
Where high workload is given as a major factor in noncompliance, an organization should think about what products it currently provides for hand hygiene. Alcohol-based hand rubs have been shown to save nursing time, which may increase overall hand hygiene compliance.[6] Organizations can make an alcohol-based hand rub available at the bedside, inside the entrance to the patient's room or in other convenient locations, as well as in individual pocket-sized containers to be carried by caregivers.

Enlist Clinical and Administrative Leader Support
Clinical and administrative leaders, whether physicians, nurses, chief executive officers, formal or informal leaders, set the tone for caregivers. Seeing these people perform hand hygiene on a regular basis encourages other professionals to follow suit and feel more comfortable speaking up

when they notice someone else neglecting such protocols. Studies have shown that when respected staff members wash their hands before touching the patients, the other staff members making rounds also wash their hands. This role modeling from the clinical setting can be extended to any setting where persons of influence can set the tone for expected behavior.[16,17]

Encourage Patient Involvement

It is important that patients realize their role in proper staff hand hygiene. Organizations should provide education to patients about hand hygiene and encourage patients and families to ask their health care providers whether they have washed their hands. Some organizations provide all staff with buttons that say, "Ask me if I've washed my hands." Sometimes, this simple question from a patient can help a provider to remember this important infection-prevention strategy. In many health care settings, patients are unlikely to challenge health care workers on this topic, so other means, such as signs in patient rooms or peer accountability, can be used to encourage hand hygiene when appropriate.

Do Not Rely on Gloves

Gloves play an important role in preventing the spread of infection but are not a substitute for hand hygiene. Many gloves have tiny perforations that allow pathogens to reach the skin. Staff might forget to remove gloves after touching one patient before moving to another. Bacteria can be spread from one part of the body to another if staff do not replace soiled gloves between tasks. Used gloves should also be removed before staff touch surfaces such as door handles or telephones. Staff should be educated about appropriate glove use, and hand washing or hand antisepsis should be carried out before and after contact with every patient, whether or not gloves are used.[18]

Ensuring the Appropriate Use of Antimicrobial Agents

Antimicrobials are used prophylactically to prevent infections and therapeutically to treat infections. Patients having surgery often receive antibiotics preoperatively and during long procedures to reduce the risk of postsurgical infections. Certain patient populations (such as those in the ICU) who are compromised with multiple or chronic illnesses, are using invasive devices, and are susceptible to infection, may receive significant quantities and several types of antimicrobials.

Antimicrobial use is complex. If antibiotics are used inappropriately, organisms can develop resistance to them, and the therapeutic usefulness of the antibiotic will decline. Many antimicrobial agents have become obsolete in this way. For some diseases and infections, there are very few antibiotics that can treat the problem successfully (for example, ventilator-associated pneumonia caused by pan-resistant *Acinetobacter baumanii*), so it is imperative to minimize resistance through appropriate use.

Case Study

Promoting Hand Hygiene
University of Geneva Hospitals

At a Glance

Organization name: University of Geneva Hospitals

City: Geneva

Country: Switzerland

Size of organization: 12,000 employees

Number of years organization has been in business: 150 years

Size of organization (number of patients, beds, etc.): 2,600 beds

Services provided and populations served: All services are provided for acute, critical, and neonatal care, and organ transplantation to rehabilitation

The Infection Control Program at the University of Geneva Hospitals, under the direction of Professor Didier Pittet, has played a leading role in the development of new strategies to promote hand hygiene. The first epidemiological study on hand hygiene was performed at the hospital in 1994. The results of this study have been the impetus of the most significant change in hand hygiene practices: the systematic recourse to alcohol-based hand rubbing as a new standard of care.

Following a baseline survey showing a compliance rate of less than 50%, a hand hygiene promotion program was started in January 1995. The most prominent component was a visual display of A3-size colour posters in 250 strategic locations that emphasized the importance of hand cleansing. Their content was prepared with collaborative groups of health care workers across all wards and translated by an artist into a cartoon-like message. Simultaneously, individual bottles of hand-rub solution were distributed in large amounts to all wards, and a newly designed flat bottle was made available to facilitate pocket carriage. Importantly, senior management supported the program that was designed as a hospitalwide priority. From the seven surveys conducted between 1994 and 1997, data were obtained on more than 20,000 opportunities for hand hygiene. Overall compliance improved from 47.6% in 1994, to 66.2% in December 1997, with a comparable increase in the use of alcohol-based hand-rub solution.

The work of Professor Pittet and his group shows clearly that strategies to improve hand hygiene must be multifaceted to be successful. They should address (a) health care worker education and motivation, (b) identification of key behavioral determinants, and (c) senior management support, which is necessary for the strategies to be fully effective. Adequate funding for hand hygiene programs is also indispensable to ensure a sustained effect on hand hygiene compliance.

(continued)

Case Study—*continued*

"Although health care–associated infections cannot be entirely eliminated, there are strategies which have been proven to be effective to reduce them significantly," Pittet says. "The fact that some health care organizations have succeeded in managing infections and the risks to patients much better than others suggests a clear patient safety improvement gap between what is possible and what is currently widely implemented."

In addition, in 2003 a new program was implemented that provided detailed descriptions of prevention measures to be applied in particular health care situations. The program described two levels of measures:

- **Basic measures** are applicable in all health care situations and, depending on the situation, involve the wearing of gloves, a mask, an apron, or protective glasses.
- **Specific measures** can complement the basic measures and must be adopted to protect a patient with reduced immune defenses or when a patient exhibits particularly dangerous infectious symptoms with a high risk of transmission, suspected or identified. In this latter case, they also serve to protect health care workers and visitors.

The introduction of a visual display notification system of the beds and wards of potentially infectious patients enables each health care worker to apply the appropriate preventive measures against infections, according to each specific situation, throughout the patient's treatment period. To ensure the correct application of measures, comprehension of the visual display notification system, and the importance of the prevention measures, the organization introduced a training program. Over nine months, 10,000 hospital workers completed a two-hour training/application session, organized in modules and provided by the Infection Control Program, in close collaboration with the training center and health care workers from other sectors of the institution.

In October 2005 the hospital took a lead role in the World Health Organization (WHO) program, "Clean Care Is Safer Care," part of the WHO's Global Patient Safety Challenge. The Global Patient Safety Challenge, a core program of the World Alliance for Patient Safety that counts Joint Commission International among its partners, has created the *WHO Guidelines on Hand Hygiene in Health Care* (Advanced Draft).

"Improved hand hygiene, a very basic and simple gesture, has the potential to reduce infections across all settings—from advanced health care systems to local dispensaries in developing countries," Pittet says. "Sometimes it's the simple things in life which bring the best results."

To ensure the proper treatment and prevention of bacterial infections, organizations should have specific policies and monitoring systems in place for antibiotic use. Antibiotic policies promote best practices, encourage or require the use of the most cost-effective drugs, and guide the prudent use of antibiotics to minimize the evolution of antibiotic-resistant strains of bacteria. If possible, a multidisciplinary oversight team or committee should design and monitor the policies. The team should include appropriate physicians and nurses, clinical pharmacist(s), microbiologist, and the infection control physician or practitioner to ensure communication between the two committees.[19] The use of decision algorithms and national or organizational guidelines to develop antibiotic use policies can be helpful. Careful use of antimicrobials through stewardship programs has been shown to reduce infections.[20,21]

After policies are created, organizations must educate practitioners about the appropriate use and administration of antibiotics. Suggestions on how to do this include the following:

- Provide educational resources such as articles and training sessions on new and existing antibiotic options.
- Provide mandatory in-services about proper use of antibiotics in surgical and nonsurgical situations. Clinical education can be effective when it is intensive, repeated, and combined with other modalities.[22]
- Engage a clinical pharmacist to make rounds with physicians. In many cases, a pharmacist can identify prescribing errors and suggest more appropriate alternatives.
- Create a restricted formulary that requires approval of restricted drugs before use. This option can be highly effective in reducing the use of targeted drugs, but may be unpopular among physicians and, in some cases, may result in the increased use of nonrestricted drugs. This can lead to incorrect prescribing patterns, antimicrobial resistance, and patient safety concerns. Restricted formularies should be reassessed often.[22]
- Provide a prophylactic antibiotic forcing function such as a dedicated nursing professional who screens all surgical patients for prophylactic antibiotics prior to surgery. This individual would determine a patient's candidacy for antibiotics and make sure that the proper medications are given.
- Develop checklists that staff can follow to make sure that appropriate considerations are given before prescribing antibiotics and that the drugs are administered in a timely manner.
- Use a computer-assisted decision system.[23] This type of system, although potentially valuable, can be quite expensive. Organizations should conduct a cost-benefit analysis on this type of system before purchasing one. These systems are not yet

available even in many well-resourced countries, but are an alternative that can be considered for the future.[24]

It is important to track antibiotic prescribing patterns and administration patterns to monitor rates and benchmark these rates against external organizations.

Ensuring Staff Health

An important part of any health care organization's IPC program is having policies in place to protect the health of its staff members. For example, every year, outbreaks of influenza cause millions of people to get sick. Health care staff are not exempt from disease and can develop influenza and other infections that, untreated, can cause significant risk to them and their patients.

One way to address this problem is to have strict policies in place that outline when an employee can and, more important, cannot report for work. For example, if an employee has an elevated temperature or infected wound, policies should dictate that he or she stays away from work until the temperature is normal for 24 hours or until the wound heals. If the employee has been exposed to chicken pox (varicella), bacterial meningitis, or tuberculosis, the organization should have policies that can be used by managers, employee health services, and the IPC team to determine tests and work guidelines to evaluate the staff and prevent exposure to others. In 1998 the US CDC published *Guidelines for Infection Control in Health Care Personnel,* which was designed to provide methods for reducing the transmission of infections from patients to health care personnel and from personnel to patients. The guidelines include recommended periods of absence from work, restrictions in the workplace, and time frames for returning to work based on the pathogen or disease.[25]

In addition to employee health policies, organizations should consider vaccinating staff for preventable communicable diseases such as influenza, measles, varicella, hepatitis A and B, and other infections relevant to infection risks in specific countries or locales. The US CDC has issued several guidelines on immunizations for health care workers in the United States, most recently on smallpox and influenza.[26,27] In some tropical countries a larger percentage of health care workers are susceptible to varicella. This increases the number of health care workers vulnerable to hospital-acquired varicella zoster virus (VZV) infection and the risk of disease transmission to coworkers and immunocompromised patients.[28] Those institutions should set policies that ensure the documentation of the VZV serostatus of all health care workers and the vaccination of susceptible ones prior to starting work. This will help limit the number of health care professionals who become ill and thus reduce the potential for the spread of infections.

Cleaning, Decontaminating, Disinfecting, or Sterilizing Equipment and Supplies

In addition to the hands of health care workers, equipment such as surgical instruments and endoscopes can transmit infection to patients.[29–34] Supplies such as bed linens can have high counts of microorganisms and serve as reservoirs for potential transmission of organisms.[35,36] Prion disease–related health risks from environmental sources of infection—including Creutzfeldt-Jakob disease (CJD), the transmission of which is linked to the use of contaminated human growth hormone, dura mater and corneal grafts, or neurosurgical equipment—are regularly fatal.[37] Individuals responsible for maintenance and repair of the equipment; cleaning, disinfection, or sterilization procedures; or laundry services are at risk for exposure to infectious organisms.

To make sure that equipment and supplies are cleaned properly, organizations should have policies and procedures in place that address at least the following issues:

- Which equipment and supplies can be cleaned and reused, as opposed to those that are disposable?
- When and how often must equipment and supplies be cleaned?
- What are the most effective cleaning, disinfection, and sterilization processes?
- How will disposable equipment that must be reused be cleaned, disinfected, or sterilized?

Nursing, IPC professionals, housekeeping and food service staff, biomedical technicians, personnel who repair and maintain equipment or clean soiled laundry, and other key staff should be involved in developing these policies. Organizations without on-site biomedical or laundry staff should nevertheless develop procedures and policies that make sure that these persons are protected from contamination and disease transmission.

Cleaning and Disinfecting Equipment

Equipment should be cleaned and disinfected before and after each patient use, as well as when it passes from one department to another. For example, all equipment should undergo appropriate decontamination before reaching an equipment maintenance department and then again before returning to the direct care environment.

Four types of processing can help remove dirt and pathogens from equipment. Depending on the type of equipment and its intended use, one of the following methods should be used to process equipment:

- Cleaning—removes all visible dust, soil, and any other visible material that microorganisms might find favorable for continued life and growth. This is usually done by scrubbing with hot water and detergent.

- Decontamination—removes disease-producing organisms, rendering equipment safe to handle
- Disinfection—destroys most disease-producing organisms but not all microbial forms. There are three levels of disinfection:
  - High level—kills all organisms except high levels of bacterial spores
  - Intermediate level—kills mycobacteria, most viruses, and bacteria
  - Low level—kills some viruses and bacteria
- Sterilization—destroys all forms of microbial life, including bacteria, viruses, spores, and fungi[38]

More than 30 years ago, E. H. Spaulding devised a classification system for determining the appropriate cleaning strategy for equipment.[39] Organizations might want to use this system to determine the category and method for decontamination of equipment. Spaulding classified items for patient care into three categories: critical, semicritical, and noncritical. These terms refer to the intended use of the device and not the potential degree of contamination. For example, the noncritical category does not imply that items cannot carry contaminants but that their degree of causing harm to health care staff and patients is not critical. Examples of each category include the following:

- **Critical.** Items in this category need to be sterilized. They include devices used to enter or come into contact with sterile tissues, such as instruments entering a surgical incision, cardiac and vascular catheters, implants, and needles placed into the vascular system.
- **Semicritical.** Items in this category generally require a high level of disinfection. These include items that come into contact with nonintact skin or mucous membranes, such as respiratory therapy equipment, anesthesia equipment, and flexible endoscopes.
- **Noncritical.** Items in this category require basic cleaning and low-level decontamination. Items that touch only intact skin would fall into this category because the skin acts as an effective barrier to most microorganisms. Such items can include crutches, bedboards, blood pressure cuffs, bedpans and urinals, and a variety of other medical accessories, as well as nonmedical accessories such as recreational equipment.

When designing policies and procedures for equipment cleaning, organizations must make sure that such policies and procedures apply to all equipment within the organization, including equipment not owned by the organization, such as demonstration, substitute, loaner, or rental units. Because such equipment moves from person to person or organization to organization and is exposed to an unknown variety of potentially infectious agents, safe practices must include appropriate cleaning of equipment before it enters and before it exits the organization, or is used on more than one patient.

Organizations can help remind staff which equipment should be cleaned, by what methods, and how frequently with noticeable, easy-to-read labels on the equipment. Checklists can be used to make sure that the appropriate staff follow all the procedures necessary to effectively clean the equipment. Logbooks that record the performance of decontamination procedures should be available and regularly monitored to make sure proper cleaning procedures are being performed. *See* Sidebar 5-2 on page 126 for more information about processing endoscopes.

Cleaning Laundry

All organizations should have a way to separate dirty from clean linen. To remove pathogens from soiled laundry such as bed sheets and gowns, the US CDC recommends that laundering be performed for a minimum of 25 minutes in at least 71°C (or 160°F) water or with chlorine bleach.[40] Laundry staff members should wash their hands after handling contaminated laundry. Food, drink, and smoking should not be permitted in the workplace.

When storing clean linen and supplies, they should be kept at least six inches off the floor so that they will not be contaminated by floor mopping. Even when linens are enclosed in plastic wrap, splash and splatter from mopping activities can contaminate the exterior surface and pose an infection risk to staff who handle them.[40]

Cleaning the Facility and Patient Environment

The environment can be a significant reservoir of microorganisms and has been implicated in transmission of health care–associated infections.[41] Therefore, in addition to equipment and supplies, organizations should address how areas of the facility will be cleaned and disinfected.[42] Cooling towers, air ventilation systems, drains, ice machines, carpeting and flooring, elevator shafts, and garbage disposal areas can all support growth of microorganisms (for example, *Legionella* and *Aspergillus*[41,43,44]). Policies and procedures should address these areas as well as equipment.

Waste Management

Contaminated waste from the health care setting can include microbiological specimens; cultures and anatomical materials; blood and body fluids from patient care activities (for example, specimens in bottles, suction containers, or units collecting body fluids); contaminated dressings, surgical drapes, and sponges; sharps, including needles, scalpel blades, and phlebotomy equipment; isolation waste from persons with highly infectious diseases such as viral hemorrhagic fevers; and other infectious materials.

Staff who manage hazardous waste are at some risk for exposure to blood and body fluids, sharps injuries, and other events. Thus, the waste must be handled and disposed of properly to prevent transmission of microorganisms to the health care staff who are containing and transporting it and

Sidebar 5-2

Processing Endoscopes

Certain types of medical equipment are more difficult to effectively clean than others. For example, endoscopes can be particularly challenging. They are used to diagnose and treat medical conditions of the gastrointestinal tract, lungs, and other sites. The incidence of infections related to endoscopes is low[1] but these devices have been linked to many health care–associated outbreaks.[2]

As with any medical device, it is important to follow the manufacturer's cleaning instructions, to train staff members carefully about cleaning methods, and to test their competency before they perform the cleaning and disinfection. One health care organization's competency review form is shown on page 127.

Although a variety of information sources discuss how to effectively clean this equipment, experts provide some helpful tips that can also be applied to other difficult-to-clean instruments:

- Clean both internal and external surfaces of the instruments with enzymatic detergent as soon as possible after use.
- Use disposable brushes for cleaning, or make sure that brushes receive high-level disinfection or sterilization. Use flushing to clean internal channels.
- Disinfect the endoscope in a high-level disinfectant or chemical sterilant making certain to reach all surfaces, channels, and crevices. A traditional agent for high-level disinfection is 2% glutaraldehyde. Newer chemical sterilants include 7.5% hydrogen peroxide, 0.08% peracetic acid plus 1.0% hydrogen peroxide, and 0.55% orthophthalaldehyde.[3]
- Rinse the endoscope with sterile water, filtered water, or tap water.
- Dry the insertion tube and channels with alcohol and forced air.
- Store the endoscope so that it dries effectively and does not become contaminated.[4]

References

1. Schembre D.B.: Infectious complications associated with gastrointestinal endoscopy. *Gastrointest Endosc Clin N Am* 10:215–232, Apr. 2000.
2. Weber D.J., Rutala W.A.: Lessons from outbreaks associated with bronchoscopy. *Infect Control Hosp Epidemiol* 22:403–408, July 2001.
3. Rutala W.A., Weber D.J.: Disinfection of endoscopes: Review of new chemical sterilants used for high-level disinfection. *Infect Control Hosp Epidemiol* 20:69–76, Jan. 1999.
4. Rutala W.A., Weber D.J.: Cleaning, disinfection and sterilization. In Pfeiffer J. (ed.): *APIC Text of Infection Control and Epidemiology.* Washington, D.C.: Association for Professionals in Infection Control and Epidemiology, Inc., 2000, pp. 55-1–55-60.

University of North Carolina Health Care System
Endoscope Reprocessing Competency

I have read the University of North Carolina Hospitals Endoscope Infection Control Policy and the Safety Policy on Glutaraldehyde Control before presenting for competency review.

Competency criteria (circle one)			Competencies
Met	Not Met	NA	Verbalizes knowledge of cleaning and disinfecting solutions used, labeling, length of effective use life, and soak times.
Met	Not Met	NA	Documents concentration of glutaraldehyde appropriately (e.g., if used daily, test daily).
Met	Not Met	NA	Wears personal protective equipment, including gown, gloves, eyewear.
Met	Not Met	NA	Demonstrates initial gross decontamination of exterior of scope and accessories. Wipes exterior of scope with clean cloth soaked in detergent or enzymatic cleaner.
Met	Not Met	NA	Leak tests scope.
Met	Not Met	NA	Uses suction to fill channels with detergent or enzymatic cleaner.
Met	Not Met	NA	Demonstrates the process of manual washing and brushing all channels, ports, and valves with appropriately prepared detergent or enzymatic cleaner.
Met	Not Met	NA	Brushes lip of biopsy port.
Met	Not Met	NA	Rinses exterior of scope, uses suction to rinse interior until fluid is clear, ends by suctioning air to clear fluid from scope.
Met	Not Met	NA	Fills interior channels with glutaraldehyde and immerses completely to prevent air bubbles. Utilizes 20-minute immersion time.
Met	Not Met	NA	Demonstrates the proper use of the automatic processor. Verbalizes knowledge of test cycles before and after use. Uses biological and chemical indicators.
Met	Not Met	NA	Avoids contaminating clean and/or disinfected items with dirty gloves. Washes hands after removing dirty gloves. Dons clean gloves prior to removing scope/accessories from glutaraldehyde.
Met	Not Met	NA	Rinses scope with sterile water, filtered water, or tap water. Uses "clean" suction.
Met	Not Met	NA	Uses forced air to dry the scope followed by alcohol to assist in drying. Then purges scope with forced air.
Met	Not Met	NA	Demonstrates proper cleaning, high-level disinfection, rinsing, and drying of all accessories.
Met	Not Met	NA	Demonstrates proper cleaning and sterilization of biopsy forceps and other cutting instruments which enter sterile body sites.
Met	Not Met	NA	Labels or packages disinfected scopes/accessories to indicate disinfection has been done.
Met	Not Met	NA	Is able to state conditions indicating a scope has not been disinfected (e.g., if not labeled or packaged, scope is considered contaminated and requires high-level disinfection prior to use).
Met	Not Met	NA	Properly stores scope/accessories in a clean location.
Met	Not Met	NA	Empties and disinfects water bottles.
Met	Not Met	NA	Disinfects brushes.
Met	Not Met	NA	Empties and cleans pans.
Met	Not Met	NA	Removes personal protective gear and discards appropriately.
Met	Not Met	NA	Washes hands before leaving reprocessing room.

I certify that this individual has met all competencies for reprocessing endoscopes.   Signature:____________________________   Date:____________
Print Name:____________________________   Title:____________

Source: North Carolina Statewide Program for Infection Control and Epidemiology (SPICE) and William A. Rutala, Ph.D., M.P.H., C.I.C. Available at http://www.unc.edu/ depts/spice/dis/Endoscope-Competency.doc. Used with permission.

SIDEBAR 5-3

Steps for Safe Management of Health Care Waste

- Assess waste production in the health care setting to determine how much is generated, what type, how often, and in what areas.
- Determine categories of waste such as general (nonrisk), hazardous, and highly hazardous.
- Evaluate treatment and disposal options in the local region—availability, effectiveness, risk to staff and environment, cost.
- Select optimal disposal option(s) for the health care setting.
- Assign responsibilities within the health care establishment, train staff, write policies and procedures, and provide protective apparel.
- Determine internal processes for waste handling by the type of waste (general health care waste clinical, infectious, hazardous), segregation and containment at the point of care, identification (labeling), transportation and storage, collection frequency, and other activities as appropriate.
- Determine processes for waste handling if transporting to an external waste management site such as a community incinerator.
- Monitor the process to ensure compliance.

---

those who are disposing of it. The most common methods to safely dispose of waste that may be considered infectious or hazardous is to incinerate it, sterilize it, or bury it in a protected landfill.

Staff who manage the waste should be trained and be provided with protective apparel such as gowns or aprons, gloves (sturdy), and, as needed, masks and eyewear. Education on the handling of sharps is particularly important because of the potential for the transmission of infections agents. Staff members involved in the disposal of sharps should also receive the appropriate vaccines and immunizations (for example, the hepatitis B vaccine). There should be systems in place for staff to report adverse events related to waste management and methods for follow-up care.[41,45–49] Steps for managing health care waste safely are listed in Sidebar 5-3 above.

Additional guidance for organizations can be found in the JCI hospital Assessment of Patients (AOP) standards, especially AOP.5.2, measurable element 3, and AOP.6.2, measurable element 4, which refer to the need to have written policies and procedures about "handling and disposal of infectious and hazardous materials" in the laboratories and in imaging suites, respectively.

Handling Food

In hospitals, long term care organizations, and other health care organizations, food and its proper handling can present a significant IPC challenge, particularly in tropical climates. When developing policies regarding food services, organizations should examine their local, regional, and national regulations and create policies that address the following:

- Proper food storage, including location, temperature, and expiration
- Proper labeling of food and nonfood items
- Procurement of food from sources that process food under regulated quality and sanitation controls
- Storage of nourishments/food items that are accessible and available for patient and family use, including food that patients or families bring from home
- Methods to prevent contamination while making, storing, and dispensing food and ice
- The use of separate or nonabsorbent and sanitized cutting boards for meat, poultry, fish, raw fruits and vegetables, and cooked foods
- Cleaning of work surfaces after each use
- Control of lighting, ventilation, and humidity to prevent moisture, condensation, and mold growth
- Appropriate employee health requirements, including the following:
  - Routine physical examinations
  - Prohibition of food preparation by an employee with an open, infected wound
  - Specific hand-washing techniques
  - Hair nets or caps and clean, washable garments
  - Absence of food, drink, or smoking in food preparation areas
- Methods for dishwashing and cleaning utensils
- Appropriate discarding of plasticware, utensils, and disposables
- Control of traffic in food service areas
- Garbage holding, transfer, and disposal

In some health care settings, families bring and prepare food for the patient. In these situations, the hospital or clinic should develop processes and guidelines that will keep the food and patients safe, including refrigeration, discarding leftover foods, washing cooking utensils, and other measures.[50]

The IPC team should be cognizant of clusters of diarrheal illnesses in staff or patients that may indicate food-borne outbreaks in the health care setting. Guidelines are available for basic food safety and for the management of these outbreaks.[51,52]

Preparing for Infection Prevention and Control Emergencies in the Health Care Setting

An IPC emergency is similar to other disasters. It is usually unexpected and unpredictable and has the potential of overwhelming an organization's care capabilities over a significant period of time. JCI standards require that all types of organizations have emergency management plans that mitigate, prepare for, respond to, and recover from emergencies. Although the Prevention and Control of Infections (PCI) standards do not specifically refer to preparation for emergencies, disasters, or catastrophes, this is an important part of any IPC program. These emergencies have implications for disease transmission from pathogens, disruptions in the environment such as floods and earthquakes, loss of basic services such as water and electricity for refrigeration, and other factors. As part of standard PCI.3, each organization should prepare for potential emergencies that could affect the health and safety of patients and increase the risk of infections. Standard FMS.10.1 requires that staff members are trained and knowledgeable about their roles in the organization's plans for fire safety, security, hazardous materials, and emergencies.

As a first step in preparing for any type of emergency, an organization's leaders should consider possible scenarios that might affect the organization and develop a plan to deal with them. The facility should be represented at emergency management meetings that involve the community. Playing the "what-if" game for each health care organization must include not only key organization staff, such as the IPC practitioner, but also representatives from the local and national sectors.

All organizations should assess their readiness and plans for in-house emergencies of many types, as described above. Although there are basic strategies that will be useful in any emergency, those related to infection risks have some specific requirements. To effectively prepare for an IPC emergency, organizations must answer many questions, including the following:

- What level of risk exists for the organization, and what response measures should be in place based on that risk? For example, a large municipal hospital in Japan may have different challenges from that of an ambulatory care clinic in India or a rural hospital in China.[53] (*See* Chapter 4's section on risk assessment.)
- Does the organization have a written plan for emergencies that can quickly be implemented and is flexible enough to respond to a variety of issues? Are the essential components of the plan easily accessible to the staff?
- How will the organization determine that an infection emergency is occurring? Who will initiate the emergency management plan?
- Are IPC professionals, emergency departments, and others monitoring the usual and unexpected infections or infection syndromes and staying informed about emerging reports from public health departments and the WHO or US CDC?
- What will the chain of command be during an emergency? How will the organization communicate effectively? How will the IPC team be notified?

- What response options are available? For example, will the organization shut down? Limit services? Restrict access? Transfer patients off site? Or will the organization act as the primary emergency facility for the community? How will special services manage patients during an emergency?[54]
- If the facility remains open, how will it manage the flow of people in and out of the building?
- If the organization must care for an unexpectedly large number of patients, how will these additional persons be accommodated—in other words, what is the organization's surge capacity?
- How will the organization deal with infected patients? If isolation is warranted, how will that be accomplished? How will the organization address the safety of patients isolated for IPC? Does the organization have adequate numbers of rooms for airborne infections or the capability to house these patients in a safe environment?[55] If appropriate, how will the organization address a mass decontamination?
- In what situations will barrier precautions be necessary? How will staff be trained on the appropriate use of those precautions? Will training incorporate both clinical and nonclinical staff?[56]
- Should quarantine or evacuation be necessary, how will it be implemented? Where will patients go? What support systems will be in place for staff? How will they be protected from acquiring or transmitting disease?
- What occupational health considerations will be necessary for staff during an emergency?
- What community resources are available? Who should be contacted and how should they be contacted? Who from the organization has this responsibility?
- How will the IPC emergency plan be integrated with the community? What community resources can work together?
- How will the plan be tested? JCI requires periodic testing of an organization's emergency management plan. It is important to test the IPC component of the plan to make sure that all issues are being addressed appropriately.

Some of the answers to these questions depend on the infectious agent involved (for example, an outbreak of smallpox warrants a different response than an influenza epidemic).

Isolating Patients During an Emergency

When an organization makes the decision to isolate a patient, it might involve placing the patient in a private room, a segregated area, or a separate building; requiring visitors and health care workers to wear protective apparel such as gowns, gloves, and masks; and restricting the movement of the patient outside of the room.[23] In some cases, visitors are restricted to limit the spread of the infection.

In the emergency management plan, organizations should identify how they will isolate large numbers of patients and make sure those patients receive prompt, safe, and documented care. Organizations isolating patients during an emergency should keep meticulous records of care to learn from the experience, share information with others, and keep track of patient and staff responses to isolation.[57]

Organizations should have a system in place to determine how supplies such as linens, eating utensils, and clothing are provided and managed for isolated patients, and they should have an emergency supply of these items in place before an influx of sick patients arrives, or have a plan to obtain them where possible. It is important for organizations to examine their current inventories of supplies, bedding, food, and water for natural disasters. When preparing for an epidemic of an infectious nature or a biological attack, looking at those inventories and determining what needs to be added would be a logical starting point.

Mass Decontamination

In the event of an IPC emergency, health care organizations might be required to remove biological residue from first responders, victims, and families. This would involve isolating the contaminated persons; decontaminating and/or treating patients; protecting staff, other patients, visitors, and the facility itself; and effectively reestablishing normal service. In preparing for this type of emergency, organizations should identify where contaminated victims will be housed, as well as how and where they will be decontaminated, regardless of the season. Organizations should also address how they will handle and store the contaminated materials.[58]

There are a few location options for decontaminating patients. Probably the most effective place is outside the main facility. By decontaminating patients in this area, organizations can protect staff, equipment, and other patients from being contaminated. If the weather is hot, tents or other temporary structures can be used to maintain privacy and keep people away from direct exposure to the elements. Decontamination showers can be set up, and individuals can be "cleaned" outside before being allowed into the facility. In this case, decontamination areas should be downwind of clean areas.[59]

Although decontaminating patients outside has its advantages, it is not always possible. In many cases, individuals enter a health care facility infected, and the organization does not know it. There is a potential that a portion of the facility itself will be contaminated and will need to be quarantined from the rest of the facility. Organizations should evaluate the layout of their facility to determine whether the air-handling systems can be isolated to prevent the spread of contaminants throughout the building and whether certain rooms, corridors, or entrances might be used to isolate or quarantine staff and patients.[58]

Equipment such as fire-rated plastic sheeting, duct tape, and spring-loaded poles can be used to cordon off hallways or other areas and separate contaminated areas from clean ones. In addition, large facilities might have decontamination rooms and showers that can be used to clean patients. Smaller organizations might determine that they are not appropriately equipped to handle emergencies involving large numbers of people and should work within the community to combine resources.[59] *See* the section "Integrating with the Community" below.

In setting up a decontamination area, there should be a "dirty" side and a "clean" side. All contaminated personnel, equipment, and victims should stay on the dirty side until decontaminated. This side should consist of a triage station, treatment station, and decontamination area. The decontamination area should accommodate both ambulatory and nonambulatory patients. Patients should perform as much of the decontamination as possible to decrease cross-contamination.

Another consideration in the mass decontamination process is the disposal of contaminated water. Runoff from showers must be controlled so that the contaminant is not tracked into clean areas. A small tub attached to each decontamination shower area can serve as a temporary holding tank, and then contaminated water can be pumped out to a larger holding area for further testing and decontamination. If a disinfectant can neutralize a biological agent, then water runoff can be allowed to go down the drain.

In addition to decontaminating patients, organizations should have a plan for decontaminating equipment. Some equipment is easy to clean and will not be too difficult to decontaminate. Others such as permanent negative air equipment will present more challenges for decontamination.

Integrating with the Community

No matter what the size of an organization, it is important to create an emergency management plan for IPC that is in harmony with the needs and resources of the community. During an IPC emergency, organizations can and should work together to identify the problem, isolate the issues, treat the patients, and return to normal operations. In creating an IPC emergency plan, organizations must meet with representatives from a variety of community agencies to make sure that any response plans capitalize on the unique strengths of the facilities and departments within the community and outline the responsibilities of those organizations. For example, organizations should meet and coordinate response plans with the following groups:

- Other health care facilities in the area, such as acute care facilities, long term care facilities, ambulatory facilities, and behavioral health care centers

- Public service organizations, such as the police and fire services, the Red Cross, hazardous materials enforcement organizations, and emergency management agencies
- Local and regional public health departments or services
- Other organizations, such as schools (including colleges and universities), churches, and community centers
- Civil defense coordinating centers
- Local and area industries and businesses
- Local and area government agencies involved with the following:
  - Housing
  - Utilities
  - Special needs populations
- Media
- Civilian groups
- Disaster-assistance nongovernmental organizations

In a communitywide effort, organizations can share resources. For example, organizations can share portable decontamination units or other buildings for childcare, communications, holding areas, alternative care sites, and showers. In addition, organizations can assist each other so that no organization is overwhelmed. For example, in a major catastrophe, Facility A could be designated as the hospital that will supply all emergency services; Facility B, which is smaller, will therefore not be overwhelmed. Facility A will transfer nonemergency patients to Facility B, send them to other local health care settings for care, or discharge them as appropriate.[58]

When developing an integrated response plan, organizations should plan the responsibilities for each organization, as well as the communication strategies between them. Following are some tips in creating such a plan:

- Include the IPC professional as an integral part of the planning, from the beginning.
- Designate a representative from each organization and department to be a member of the overall emergency coordinating body.
- Make sure that each organization maintains its own emergency response plan (for example, a health center may have a different plan from the acute care hospital).
- Identify to whom information about the emergency should be communicated, including public health organizations and a multiorganizational emergency management team.
- Designate multiple means of communication in case standard methods are unavailable. For example, should phone or fax systems become disabled, organizations should have plans to use radio technology or wireless and Internet communication.

- Determine how temporary credentialing and privileging policies will be assigned so that personnel can "float" between organizations if necessary.
- State to whom any volunteers are to report and outline a clear line of supervision.
- Identify ways of transporting patients to and from different facilities.

No one knows when, where, and whether a biological emergency will occur, but all organizations should take the time to effectively plan for one. Addressing issues of identification, isolation, and decontamination, as well as identifying the resources within a community will help organizations to preserve the safety of patients and the community as a whole.

Conclusion

This chapter has described some of the ongoing efforts to maintain and continually improve the IPC program. Continual vigilance about IPC practices, new science, and updated recommendations are critical to this effort. It is incumbent on the IPC team to look for new ways to reduce infections, review the literature, evaluate implementation of policies, and involve leadership. These efforts will go far in improving patient safety and the quality of care in any health care setting.

References

1. Joint Commission Resources: Infection control: Covering all the bases. *Joint Commission Benchmark* 6:1,9, Mar.–Apr. 2004.
2. van Tiel F.H., et al.: Plan-do-study-act cycles as an instrument for improvement of compliance with infection control measures in care of patients after cardiothoracic surgery. *J Hosp Infect* 62:64–70, Jan. 2006.
3. Gering J., et al.: Taking a patient safety approach to an integration of two hospitals. *Jt Comm J Qual Patient Saf* 31:258–266, May 2005.
4. Eldridge N.E., et al.: Using the six sigma process to implement the Centers for Disease Control and Prevention Guideline for Hand Hygiene in 4 intensive care units. *J Gen Intern Med* 21 (suppl. 2):S35–S42, Feb. 2006.
5. Arias K.: Surveillance. In Carrick R. (ed.): *APIC Text of Infection Control and Epidemiology,* 2nd ed. Washington, D.C.: Association for Professionals in Infection Control and Epidemiology, Inc., 2005.
6. Centers for Disease Control and Prevention: *Hand Hygiene Guidelines Fact Sheet.* 2002. http://www.cdc.gov/od/oc/media/pressrel/fs021025.htm (accessed Apr. 19, 2006).
7. World Health Organization (WHO): *WHO Guidelines on Hand Hygiene in Health Care* (Advanced Draft): *A Summary.* Geneva: WHO, 2005.
8. Rutala B., et al.: Disinfection of computer keyboards. *Infect Control Hosp Epidemiol* 27:372–377, Apr. 2006.

9. Lankford M.G., et al.: Assessment of materials commonly utilized in health care: Implications for bacterial survival and transmission. *Am J Infect Control* 34:258–263, Jun. 2006.

10. Brady R.R., et al.: Is your phone bugged? The incidence of bacteria known to cause nosocomial infection on healthcare workers' mobile phones. *J Hosp Infect* 62(1):123–125, Jan. 2006.

11. Institute for Healthcare Improvement: *100k Lives Campaign.* 2006. http://www.ihi.org/IHI/Programs/Campaign (accessed Jul. 11, 2006).

12. Pittet D.: Improving adherence to hand hygiene practice: A multidisciplinary approach. *Emerg Infect Dis* 7:234–240, Mar.–Apr. 2001.

13. Larson E.: State-of-the-science—2004: Time for a "No Excuses/No Tolerance" (NET) strategy. *Am J Infect Control* 33:548–557, Nov. 2005.

14. Larson E.L., et al.: An organizational climate intervention associated with increased handwashing and decreased nosocomial infections. *Behav Med* 26(1):14–22, 2000.

15. Pittet D., et al.: Hand hygiene among physicians: Performance, beliefs, and perceptions. *Ann Intern Med* 141:1–8, Jul. 6, 2004.

16. Snow M., et al.: Mentor's hand hygiene practices influence student's hand hygiene rates. *Am J Infect Control* 34:18–24, Feb. 2006.

17. Lankford M.G., et al.: Influence of role models and hospital design on hand hygiene of healthcare workers. *Emerg Infect Dis* 9:217–223, Feb. 2003.

18. Larson E.: [Handwashing: It is essential even when gloves are used]. [Article in Portuguese]. *Servir* 38:275–279, Nov.–Dec. 1990.

19. Principles of Antibiotic Policy. In French G., Friedman C. (eds.): *Infection Control: Basic Concepts and Practices.* 2nd ed. International Federation of Infection Control. 2003. http://www.theific.org/oldsite/Manual/toc.htm.

20. Fishman N.: Antimicrobial stewardship. *Am J Med* 119 (suppl. 1):S53–S61; discussion S62–S70, Jun. 2006.

21. Paskovaty A., et al.: A multidisciplinary approach to antimicrobial stewardship: Evolution into the 21st century. *Int J Antimicrob Agents* 25:1–10, Jan. 2005.

22. Schwartz D.: Errant antibiotic use: Consequences and improvement potential. Paper presented at the Joint Commission on Accreditation of Healthcare Organization's Infection Control Conference, Chicago, Nov. 17, 2003.

23. Stelfox H., Bates D.: Safety of patients isolated for infection control. *JAMA* 290:1899–1905, Oct. 8, 2003.

24. Thursky K.: Use of computerized decision support systems to improve antibiotic prescribing. *Expert Rev Anti Infect Ther* 4:491–507, Jun. 2006.

25. Centers for Disease Control and Prevention: *Guidelines for Infection Control in Health Care Personnel.* 1998. http://www.cdc.gov/ncidod/dhqp/ gl_hcpersonnel.html (accessed Jul. 11, 2006).

26. Wharton M., et al.; Advisory Committee on Immunization Practices; Healthcare Infection Control Practices Advisory Committee: Recommendations for using smallpox vaccine in a pre-event vaccination program. Supplemental recommendations of the Advisory Committee on Immunization Practices (ACIP) and the Healthcare Infection Control Practices Advisory Committee (HICPAC). *MMWR Recomm Rep* 52:1–16, Apr. 4, 2003.

27. Centers for Disease Control and Prevention: Prevention and control of influenza: Recommendations of the Advisory Committee on Immunization Practices (ACIP). *MMWR* 54:1–40, Jul. 29, 2005.

28. Almuneef M., et al.: Varicella zoster virus immunity in multinational health care workers of a Saudi Arabian hospital. *Am J Infect Control* 31:375–381, Oct. 2003.

29. Srinivasan A., et al.: An outbreak of *Pseudomonas aeruginosa* infections associated with flexible bronchoscopes. *N Engl J Med* 348:221–227, Jan. 16, 2003.

30. Fraser T.G., et al.: Multidrug-resistant *Pseudomonas aeruginosa* cholangitis after endoscopic retrograde cholangiopancreatography: Failure of routine endoscope cultures to prevent an outbreak. *Infect Control Hosp Epidemiol* 25:856–859, Oct. 2004.

31. Cetre J.C., et al.: Outbreaks of contaminated broncho-alveolar lavage related to intrinsically defective bronchoscopes. *J Hosp Infect* 61:39–45, Sep. 2005.

32. Corne P., et al.: Unusual implication of biopsy forceps in outbreaks of *Pseudomonas aeruginosa* infections and pseudo-infections related to bronchoscopy. *J Hosp Infect* 61:20–26, Sep. 2005.

33. Kibria S.M., et al.: Bacterial colonisation of Doppler probes on vascular surgical wards. *Eur J Vasc Endovasc Surg* 23:241–243, Mar. 2002.

34. Swaddiwudhipong W., et al.: A report of an outbreak of postoperative endophthalmitis. *J Med Assoc Thai* 83:902–907, Aug. 2000.

35. Barrie D., et al.: Bacillus cereus meningitis in two neurosurgical patients: An investigation into the source of the organism. *J Infect* 25:291–297, Nov. 1992.

36. Ndawula E.M., Brown L.: Mattresses as reservoirs of epidemic methicillin-resistant *Staphylococcus aureus*. *Lancet* 337:488, Feb. 23, 1991.

37. Rutala W.A., Weber, D.J.: Cleaning, disinfection and sterilization. In Pfeiffer J. (ed.): *APIC Text of Infection Control and Epidemiology*. Washington, D.C.: Association for Professionals in Infection Control and Epidemiology, Inc., 2000, pp. 55-1–55-60.

38. Spaulding E.H.: Chemical disinfection of medical and surgical materials. In Lawrence C.A., Block S.S. (eds.): *Disinfection, Sterilization and Preservation*. Philadelphia: Lea and Febiger, 1968, pp. 517–531.

39. Centers for Disease Control and Prevention: *Guidelines for Laundry in Health Care Facilities*. 2002. http://www.cdc.gov/od/ohs/biosfty/laundry.htm (accessed Mar. 14, 2006).

40. Sehulster L., Chinn R.Y.; CDC; HICPAC. Guidelines for environmental infection control in health-care facilities: Recommendations of CDC and the Healthcare Infection Control Practices Advisory Committee (HICPAC). *MMWR Recomm Rep* 52:1–42, Jun. 6, 2003.

41. Rutala W.A., Weber D.J.: The benefits of surface disinfection. *Am J Infect Control* 33:434–435, Sep. 2005.

42. Lass-Florl C., et al.: Epidemiology and outcome of infections due to *Aspergillus terreus*: 10-year single centre experience. *Br J Haematol* 131:201–207, Oct. 2005.

43. Warris A., Verweij P.E.: Clinical implications of environmental sources for *Aspergillus*. *Med Mycol* 43 (suppl. 1):S59–S65, May 2005.

44. Prüss A., Giroult E., Rushbrook P. (eds.): *WHO Safe Management of Wastes from Healthcare Activities*. World Health Organization. 1999. http://www.who.int/water_sanitation_health/medicalwaste/167to180.pdf (accessed Jul. 12, 2006).

45. Infection Control. In French G., Friedman C. (eds.): *Infection Control: Basic Concepts and Practices.* 2nd ed. International Federation of Infection Control. 2003. http://www.theific.org/oldsite/Manual/toc.htm (accessed Jul. 10, 2006).
46. Djeriri K., et al.: [Occupational risk for blood exposure and staff behaviour: A cross-sectional study in 3 Moroccan healthcare centers] [Article in French]. *Med Mal Infect* 35:396–401, Jul.–Aug. 2005.
47. Massrouje H.T.: Medical waste and health workers in Gaza governorates. *East Mediterr Health J* 7:1017–1024, Nov. 2001.
48. Akter N., et al.: Hospital waste management and its probable health effect: A lesson learned from Bangladesh. *Indian J Environ Health* 44:124–137, Apr. 2002.
49. World Health Organziation: *Basic Food Safety for Health Workers.* 1999. http://www.who.int/foodsafety/publications/capacity/healthworkers/en/ (accessed Jul. 6, 2006).
50. Reglier-Poupet H., et al.: Evaluation of the quality of hospital food from the kitchen to the patient. *J Hosp Infect* 59:131–137, Feb. 2005.
51. Department of Health (UK): *Management of outbreaks of food borne illness.* London: Department of Health, 1994.
52. Imai T., et al.: Substantial differences in preparedness for emergency infection control measures among major hospitals in Japan: Lessons from SARS. *J Infect Chemother* 12:124–131, Jun. 2006.
53. Lin Y.C., et al.: Emergency management and infection control in a radiology department during an outbreak of severe acute respiratory syndrome. *Br J Radiol* 78:606–611, Jul. 2005.
54. Rebmann T.: Management of patients infected with airborne-spread diseases: An algorithm for infection control professionals. *Am J Infect Control* 33:571–579, Dec. 2005.
55. Filoromo C., et al.: An innovative approach to training hospital-based clinicians for bioterrorist attacks. *Am J Infect Control* 31:511–514, Dec. 2003.
56. Oren M.: Quarantine after an international biological weapons attack: Medical and public health requirements for containment. *Isr Med Assoc J* 6:658–660, Nov. 2004.
57. Hammond J.: Mass casualty incidents: Planning implications for trauma care. *Scand J Surg* 94(4):267–271, 2005.
58. Braun B.I., et al.: Integrating hospitals into community emergency preparedness planning. *Ann Intern Med* 144:799–811, Jun. 6, 2006.
59. Joint Commission Resources: *Standing Together: An Emergency Planning Guide for America's Communities.* Oakbrook Terrace, IL: Joint Commission on Accreditation of Healthcare Organizations, 2004.

Further Readings

Boyce J., Pittet D.: Guideline for hand hygiene in health-care settings. *MMWR* 51(RR-16):1–45, 2002.
Burke J.P.: Infection control—A problem for patient safety. *N Engl J Med* 348:651–656, Feb. 13, 2003.
Buso D.L., et al.: Development and organisation of an instructional course on epidemic/outbreak preparedness and response for health workers in the Eastern Cape. *S Afr Med J* 95:932–933, 936–937, Dec. 2005.
Centers for Disease Control and Prevention: *Immunization of Healthcare Workers.* http://www.cdc.gov/ncidod/dhqp/wrkr_immune.html.

Cleaning, disinfection and sterilization. In French G., Friedman C. (eds.): *Infection Control: Basic Concepts and Practices*. 2nd ed. International Federation of Infection Control. 2003. http://www.theific.org/oldsite/Manual/toc.htm.

Coles G., et al.: Using failure mode effects and criticality analysis for high-risk processes at three community hospitals. *Joint Commission Journal on Quality and Patient Safety* 31:132–140, Mar. 2005.

French G.L.: Antimicrobial resistance in hospital flora and nosocomial infections. In: Mayhall C.G. (ed.): *Hospital Epidemiology and Infection Control*, 3rd ed. Philadelphia: Lippincott Williams & Wilkins, 2004, pp.1613–1638.

Handwashing Liaison Group: Handwashing: A modest measure with big effects. *BMJ* 318:686, Mar. 1999.

Ippolito G., et al.: Hospital preparedness and management of patients affected by viral haemorrhagic fever or smallpox at the Lazzaro Spallanzani Institute, Italy. *Euro Surveill* 10:36–39, Mar. 2005.

Joint Commission Resources: *Failure Mode and Effects Analysis in Health Care: Proactive Risk Reduction*, 2nd ed. Oakbrook Terrace, IL: Joint Commission on Accreditation of Healthcare Organizations, 2005.

———: *Root Cause Analysis in Health Care: Tools and Techniques*, 3rd ed. Oakbrook Terrace, IL: Joint Commission on Accreditation of Healthcare Organizations, 2005.

———: Systems analysis: Prioritizing processes for FMEA. *Joint Commission Perspectives on Patient Safety* 5:7–8, May 2005.

Kimchi-Woods J., Shultz J.P.: Using HFMEA to assess potential for patient harm from tubing misconnections. *Joint Commission Journal on Quality and Patient Safety* 32:373–381, Jul. 2006.

MacDougall C., Polk R.E.: Antimicrobial stewardship programs in health care systems. *Clin Microbiol Rev* 18:638–656, Oct. 2005.

Mills, P.D., et al.: Using aggregate root cause analysis to reduce falls and related injuries. *Joint Commission Journal on Quality and Patient Safety* 31:21–31, Jan. 2005.

Occupational health risks for health care workers. In French G., Friedman C. (eds.): *Infection Control: Basic Concepts and Practices*. 2nd ed. International Federation of Infection Control. 2003. http://www.theific.org/oldsite/Manual/toc.htm.

Rebmann, T.: Disaster management. In: Carrick R. (ed.): *APIC Text of Infection Control and Epidemiology*. Washington D.C.: Assocation of Professionals in Infection Control and Epidemiology, Inc., 2005.

Shadel B.N., et al.: What we need to know about bioterrorism preparedness: Results from focus groups conducted at APIC 2000. *Am J Infect Control* 29:347–351, Dec. 2001.

Shadel B.N., et al.: Infection control practitioners' perceptions and educational needs regarding bioterrorism: Results from a national needs assessment survey. *Am J Infect Control* 31:129–134, May 2003.

Resources

The following readings were gathered for use in *Information Resources in Infection Control,* Fourth Edition (Editor: Nizam Damani M.D., MBBS, MSc, FRCPI, FRCPath), due in 2006 from the International Federation of Infection Control (IFIC). The full document will be available online at IFIC's Web site: http://www.theific.org/publications.asp. NOTE: Some of these resources may appear at the end of more than one chapter, due to their applicability to more than one aspect of infection prevention and control.

American Thoracic Society and the Infectious Diseases Society of America: Guidelines for the management of adults with hospital-acquired, ventilator-associated, and healthcare-associated Pneumonia. *Am J Respir Crit Care Med* 171:388–416, Feb. 2005.

Association for Professionals in Infection Control and Epidemiology, Inc.: APIC Surveillance Initiative Working Group. Recommended practice for surveillance. *Am J Infect Control* 26:277–288, Jun. 1998.

Association for Professionals in Infection Control and Epidemiology, Inc.: APIC Surveillance Initiative Working Group. Recommended practice for surveillance. *Am J Infect Control* 26:277–288, Jun. 1998.

Centers for Disease Control and Prevention: Guidelines for prevention of nosocomial pneumonia. *MMWR Morb Mortal Wkly Rep* 46(RR-1):1–79, 1997. http://www.cdc.gov/mmwr/preview/mmwrhtml/00045365.htm.

———: CDC definitions of surgical sites infections, 1992: A modification of the CDC definitions of wound infections. *Am J Infect Control* 20:271–274, Oct. 1992.

Cruse P.J.E., Foord R.: The epidemiology of wound infections: A 10-year prospective study of 62,939 wounds. *Surg Clin North Am* 60:27–40, Feb. 1980.

———: A five-year prospective study of 23,649 surgical wounds. *Arch Surg* 107:206–210, Aug. 1973.

Department of Health (UK): Guidelines for preventing infections associated with the insertion and maintenance central venous catheters. *J Hosp Infect* 47 (suppl.): S47–S67, Oct. 2001. http://www.dh.gov.uk/assetRoot/04/07/73/68/04077368.PDF.

Department of Health (UK): Guidelines for preventing infections associated with the insertion and maintenance of short-term indwelling urethral catheters in acute care. *J Hospl Infect* 47 (suppl.):S39–S46, Oct. 2001.

Emmerson A.M., et al.: The Second National Prevalence Survey of Infection in Hospitals—Overview of the results. *J Hosp Infect* 32:175–190, Jan. 1996.

Gaynes R.P., et al.: Surgical site infection (SSI) rates in the United States, 1992–1998: The NNIS basic risk index. *Clin Infect Dis* 33 (suppl. 2):S78–S63, Sep. 2001.

Glenister H.M., et al.: *A Study of Surveillance Methods for Detecting Hospital Infection.* London: Public Health Laboratory Service, 1992.

Glynn A., et al.: *Hospital-Acquired Infection: Surveillance, Policies and Practice.* London: Public Health Laboratory Service, 1997.

Haley R.W., et al.: The efficacy of infection surveillance and control programs in preventing nosocomial infection in US hospitals (SENIC study). *Am J Epidemiol* 121(2):182–205, 1985.

Health Protection Agency (UK): *Protocol for Surveillance of Surgical Site Infection.* 2004. www.hpa.org.uk/.

Hospital Infection Society (UK): Behaviours and rituals in the operating theatre. *J Hosp Infect* 51:241–255, Aug. 2002. http://www.his.org.uk/_db/_documents/OTIC-final.pdf.

Infection Control Nurses Association (ICNA): *Guidelines for Preventing Intravascular Catheter-Related Infection.* Bathgate, UK: ICNA, 2001.

Klaucke D.N., et al.: Guidelines for evaluating surveillance systems. *MMWR Morb Mortal Wkly Rep* 37(suppl. 5):1–18, May 1988. http://www.cdc.gov/mmwr/preview/mmwrhtml/00001769.htm.

Mangram A., et al. CDC guideline for prevention of surgical site infection. *Infect Control Hosp Epidemiol* 20(4):247–280, 1999.

McGeer A., et al.: Definitions of infection for surveillance in long term care facilities. *Am J Infect Control* 19(1):1–7, 1991.

Mermel L.A., et al.: Guidelines for the management of intravascular catheter-related infections. *Clin Infect Dis* 32(9):1249–1272, 2001.

Nicolle L.E.: Urinary tract infections in long-term-care facilities (SHEA Position Paper). *Infect Control Hosp Epidemiol* 22:167–175, Sep. 2001.

Public Health Agency of Canada: Preventing infections associated with indwelling intravascular access devices. *Can Commun Dis Rep* 23S8, Sep. 1997.

Public Health Laboratory Service (PHLS): *Socioeconomic Burden of Hospital-Acquired Infection.* London: PHLS, 1999.

Tablan O.C., et al., Centers for Disease Control and Prevention: Guidelines for preventing healthcare associated pneumonia, 2003. *MMWR Morb Mortal Wkly Rep* 53(RR-03):1–36, 2004. http://www.cdc.gov/mmwr/preview/mmwrhtml/rr5303a1.htm.

CHAPTER SIX

Lessons Learned
The 2003 Hong Kong and Toronto SARS Outbreaks

In November 2002 severe acute respiratory syndrome (SARS) was first recognized in the Guangdong Province of China.[1] This syndrome was characterized by fever, headache, myalgia, cough, and shortness of breath. It led to pneumonia and occasionally to acute respiratory distress and death.[2] By February 2003 SARS had spread to Hong Kong, and on February 23 the disease crossed the world and arrived in Toronto, Canada. The Hong Kong outbreak resulted in 1,755 cases of SARS and 299 deaths.[3] The Toronto outbreak occurred in two phases that resulted in 389 cases of SARS and 44 deaths.[4,5]

The experiences of Hong Kong and Toronto with SARS provide an opportunity to see how health delivery systems can falter during a crisis involving an emerging or reemerging infection. The responses of Hong Kong and Canada to the disease offer lessons as to what health care organizations did well and what they did not. The purpose of this chapter is to outline the progression of SARS in these two major cities and offer some lessons that health care organizations can apply to their infection prevention and control (IPC) programs.

Phase One

Examining each of the cases in Hong Kong and Toronto would exceed the scope of this book, but it is helpful to review a few cases to see how quickly and how far a disease can spread when it is initially left unchecked. Following is a discussion of some of the Hong Kong and Toronto cases and how they affected one another. (*See* Sidebar 6-1 on page 144 for a time line of the SARS outbreaks and Sidebar 6-2 on page 147 for information on how SARS spread in Hong Kong.)

Hong Kong Outbreak

Hong Kong's location along the border with China and its massive population in a very compact city made it particularly vulnerable to the SARS

Sidebar 6-1

A SARS Time Line

November 2002—The first known case of SARS occurs in Guangdong Province, China; the actual SARS virus is not identified, though, until many months later.

10 February 2003—The Beijing office of the World Health Organization (WHO) learns that more than 100 people are dead from a new contagious disease that is causing panic in Guangdong Province.

10–14 February 2003—Guangdong Province reports more than 300 cases and 5 deaths. The Chinese Ministry of Health tells the WHO that this is an outbreak of atypical pneumonia that is coming under control.

17–20 February 2003—A Hong Kong man dies after traveling to China the month before; his daughter died previously, and his son is sick with what is reported to be the A (H5N1) influenza virus—the virus also identified as having infected the father.

21–25 February 2003—The illness begins to spread as a physician from Guangdong Province attends a wedding in Hong Kong, staying in a hotel and later seeking treatment at the city's Kwong Wah Hospital. A Toronto woman stays at the same Hong Kong hotel as the infected physician before returning home to Canada. During this same time, a man who visited the same hotel becomes sick and a Hong Kong–based relative of the Guangdong Province physician seeks treatment at Kwong Wah Hospital.

4 March 2003—The Guangdong Province physician dies at Kwong Wah Hospital in Hong Kong.

7 March 2003—Health care workers at Prince of Wales Hospital in Hong Kong become sick with what is believed to be a form of pneumonia.

12 March 2003—The WHO issues a global alert about cases of severe atypical pneumonia.

14 March 2003—Health care workers at three hospitals in Hong Kong show signs of pneumonia. Canadian officials announce that four cases of atypical pneumonia have been reported in Toronto.

15 March 2003—The WHO names the illness severe acute respiratory syndrome (SARS) and issues an international travel advisory.

18–19 March 2003—Hong Kong reports more than 120 cases, and analysis shows that most are occurring in health care workers or those having close contact with infected individuals. The brother-in-law of Guangdong Province physician dies in a Hong Kong hospital.

30 March 2003—Hong Kong health officials publicly identify the Amoy Gardens housing complex as the site of a SARS outbreak, with 213 residents hospitalized.

2 April 2003—The WHO issues an alert advising against all but essential travel to Hong Kong and Guangdong Province, representing the strongest travel advisory ever issued by the WHO.

SIDEBAR 6-1—CONTINUED

16 April 2003—The WHO announces that SARS is the result of a coronavirus that is unlike any human or animal strain identified in the past.

23 April 2003—The WHO extends the travel advisory to include Toronto, as well as Beijing and Shanxi Province in China.

30 April 2003—The WHO lifts the travel advisory for Toronto.

7 May 2003—The WHO estimates that 14% to 15% of patients with SARS die.

22 May 2003—Toronto officials report new cases of acute respiratory illness.

23 May 2003—The WHO lifts travel advisories for Hong Kong and Guangdong Province.

26 May 2003—The WHO adds Toronto once again to the list of areas with recent local SARS transmissions.

23 June 2003—The WHO removes Hong Kong from the SARS transmissions list.

5 July 2003—The WHO declares containment of the worldwide SARS outbreak.

Source: World Health Organization: *Update 95—SARS: Chronology of a serial killer.* 2003. http://www.who.int/csr/don/2003_07_04/en/.

outbreak that flourished in early 2003. Reports of the rapid spread of a new respiratory disease in the Guangdong Province of China caught the attention of the media in February 2003, prompting the Hong Kong Department of Health, as well as a team of experts from the World Health Organization (WHO), to observe efforts to identify and contain the illness. The Hong Kong Hospital Authority further stepped up monitoring by establishing a surveillance system for cases of atypical pneumonia in public hospitals. [6]

During this same period of mid-February and early March 2003, the system identified the case of a physician from China with severe community-acquired pneumonia. The physician had stayed at a Hong Kong hotel while visiting family members and was admitted a short time later to Kwong Wah Hospital. Subsequent epidemiology studies showed that nine other people, including health care workers, who either were in close contact with the man or stayed at the same Hong Kong hotel became ill. These individuals included the physician's brother-in-law, a Hong Kong resident who had spent most of a day with the infected man; a nurse who had no direct contact with the infected physician other than being present in the same hospital treatment area as this index patient; a Chinese man visiting Hong Kong and staying at the same hotel as the infected physician; a health care assistant who came into contact with the physician's infected brother-in-law in the intensive care unit (ICU) of the hospital; three nurses who worked at the hospital where the Chinese man visiting Hong Kong and staying at the hotel eventually sought treatment; the nephew of the Chinese man visiting Hong Kong and staying at the hotel; and a patient who stayed in the same hospital area as the Chinese man visiting Hong Kong and staying at the hotel.[7] The Chinese physician identified as the index patient and his brother-in-law both died.

An Epidemic in Hong Kong

The first realization that Hong Kong might be facing an epidemic did not occur until 10 March 2003, with the report of an outbreak of respiratory infections involving 11 staff members from Prince of Wales Hospital. All of the health care workers were from the same ward, prompting hospital officials to immediately close the area to new patients and to outside visitors.[6] Prince of Wales Hospital eased the visiting policy for the ward the next day to require that anyone coming into the ward had to be protected by surgical masks, disposable gloves, and disposable gowns.

The index patient in the Prince of Wales Hospital outbreak was actually hospitalized on 4 March 2003, and the disease began spreading to others at the facility over the next four days as the man was treated in the general medical area of the facility. Authorities later discovered that this man had been a visitor at the Hong Kong hotel where the infected Chinese physician in the first known Hong Kong outbreak had been a guest. Hong Kong health officials eventually would link more than 100 cases of infection to contact with this Prince of Wales Hospital index patient. [8]

Amoy Gardens Outbreak

Late in March 2003, Hong Kong officials discovered that another outbreak was occurring in the city. This time, however, the outbreak was at a residential complex. The index patient in this wave of SARS in Hong Kong had stayed at the Amoy Gardens apartments for a night in mid-March and was admitted to Prince of Wales Hospital the next day with symptoms of atypical pneumonia.[6] By the end of the month, more than 300 residents at Amoy Gardens were affected. [9]

Toronto Case A

From 13 through 23 February 2003, a 78-year-old Chinese woman from Canada traveled with her husband to Hong Kong to visit family. For 4 of the 10 days she stayed at the Metropole Hotel in Kowloon.[1] Unbeknownst to her, a Chinese physician who had SARS was staying at the same hotel. The irony is that the Canadian woman didn't need to stay in the hotel at all because she was in Hong Kong to see family and could have stayed with them. However, the hotel was part of a package deal.[10]

On 23 February 2003, the woman returned to Toronto and subsequently developed a fever, anorexia, myalgias, a sore throat, and a mild productive

---

How SARS Spread in Hong Kong

The outbreak of SARS in Hong Kong led to many questions about how the infection spread, particularly whether more could have been done to stop the progression. A follow-up study of patients with probable SARS showed the following:

- 26.6% worked at hospitals
- 16.1% had secondary infections as the result of living in the same household as SARS patients
- 14.3% lived at the Amoy Gardens housing complex
- 9.9% came into contact with nonfamily SARS patients as the result of interactions in the community or health care settings
- 4.9% were inpatients

The source of infection could not be determined for 29.1% of those studied. Researchers seeking to link these cases to the SARS outbreak were able to find a number of common factors, including visits to mainland China, Amoy Gardens, Prince of Wales Hospital, or other facilities that treated infected patients. Further analysis revealed that 44% of these cases involved people who had some sort of connection to a hospital where SARS patients were treated. The connections ranged from health care workers to inpatients to visitors. Combined with information about the number of health care workers and inpatients who developed SARS, this shows the importance of preventing and controlling health care–associated infections.

Source: Lau J.T.F., et al.: SARS transmission, risk factors, and prevention in Hong Kong. *Emerg Infect Dis* 10, Apr. 2004. http://www.cdc.gov/ncidod/EID/vol10no4/03-0628.htm (accessed Apr. 19, 2006).

cough. Her condition deteriorated and she subsequently died at home on March 5.[1,2] This woman became Toronto's index case (Case A) for SARS.

Toronto Case B

When she was ill, Case A spread the infection to those family members who cared for her. One of the family members who became ill was her son (Case B). On 7 March 2003, he visited the emergency room (ER) of Scarborough Grace Hospital, a community hospital located in an eastern suburb of Toronto. Case B arrived at Scarborough Grace before the WHO issued its alert about SARS and initiated global surveillance. Because the hospital was unaware of SARS, Case B was placed in a general observation area of the ER with only curtains separating patients. He received management of his respiratory symptoms, including nebulized salbutamol.[1,2] During this time, SARS was transmitted from Case B to two other patients in the ER general observation area (Cases C and D).[1] Case C was in the bed adjacent to Case B about 1.5 meters away. He remained in the ER for nine hours and then was discharged home.[2] Case D was three beds away from Case B and was transferred to a hospital ward and later discharged home on 10 March. The three patients were cared for by the same nurse.[2]

On 13 March 2003, Case B died. It was then that public health officials first realized that Toronto had a case of SARS. This was also the day after the WHO issued its global alert. Scarborough Grace Hospital implemented airborne, contact, and droplet precautions for staff caring for known cases of SARS, which at the time were Case B and members of his family who had come to visit him on 8, 9, and 10 March.[2]

On 13 March, four of Case B's family members were admitted to three different hospitals, and a fifth family member was admitted the following day. All of these cases were managed using airborne, droplet, and contact precautions, and SARS did not further progress from these cases after their admission to the hospitals.[2] In the end, 6 of the 11 members of Case A's family became infected and two died.[1]

Toronto Case C

Three days after meeting Case B in the ER, Case C began exhibiting symptoms of SARS. On 16 March 2003, he was brought back to the hospital. After nine hours in the ER where airborne, contact, and droplet precautions were used, he was transferred into the ICU and placed in isolation. His wife became ill on 16 March. She was with him in the ER on that day and visited him in the ICU on 21 March 2003. Later that day, he died.[2] She also succumbed to SARS after a few days. Following is a list of the individuals whom Case C and his wife infected before they succumbed:

- Three other members of their household
- The two paramedics and one firefighter who transported Case C to the hospital
- Five ER staff, one other hospital staff, and one housekeeper who worked in the ER while Case C was there
- The ICU physician who intubated Case C. This individual wore a surgical mask, gown, and gloves when performing the procedure. The physician transmitted the infection to one member of his family. Three ICU nurses who were present at the intubation had onset of early symptoms between 18 and 20 March. One of these nurses transmitted the infection to a household member.
- Two patients and seven visitors who were in the ER at the same time as Case C's wife. The seven ER visitors gave the infection to five household members and other family contacts.[1,2]

On the evening of 16 March 2003, the elderly grandfather of a large family was taken to Scarborough Grace Hospital for an injured knee.[1,10] Case C and his wife were there. The grandfather and two members of his family who were with him contracted SARS. On 1 April 2003, the grandfather died and symptomatic family members were present at his funeral.[1] In addition, the family was part of a religious group that engaged in frequent worship and social activities. This group held two large events during the latter part of March. The first event was attended by 500 people, and 250 were registered for the second.[1] The virus began to spread among members of this group. For a time, it appeared that SARS would spread in an untraceable and uncontrollable fashion. Fortunately, it did not; however, by the time this cluster was contained, 14 members of the grandfather's family, 14 members of the religious group, and 3 health care workers were infected.[10]

By 22 March 2003, Scarborough Grace Hospital was implementing contact and droplet precautions for all patients in the ICU, and the ICU and emergency departments were closed on 23 March. The next day, following the identification of staff and patient cases not linked to the ICU or ER, the hospital was closed to admissions, outpatient clinics were closed, and discharged patients were placed into quarantine at home for 10 days.[2] Active surveillance for SARS was established.[1]

By the end of Phase One, 129 cases of SARS stemmed from Scarborough Grace Hospital. Approximately 85 households were involved, and SARS was transmitted to 25% of those households.[1]

Toronto Case D

On 13 March 2003, Case D became ill and was brought to Scarborough Grace by emergency medical services (EMS) personnel. Because he presented with a myocardial infarction and staff did not know that he had contact with Case B, it was not recognized that he had SARS, and standard IPC precautions were not used. He remained in the cardiac care unit (CCU) for three days and was then transferred to another hospital for renal dialysis. Before being transferred, Case D transmitted the infection to one patient in the ER, three emergency department staff, one housekeeper who worked in the ER while Case D was there, one physician, two hospital technologists, two CCU patients, seven CCU staff, and one EMS paramedic who transported Case D to the hospital. These individuals then transmitted the disease to six of their family members, one patient, one medical clinical staff, and one other nurse in the emergency department.[1, 2]

When Case D was transferred, he again was not put under any special isolation procedures. On 21 March 2003, his wife was admitted to the surgical unit of the hospital with fractured ribs. It is believed that the couple was the source of this hospital's outbreak. After the couple was admitted to the hospital, the organization identified five staff members who had SARS. The organization began strict droplet IPC precautions throughout the hospital. One of the infected staff members worked as a dialysis nurse and had worked a shift while exhibiting symptoms. Follow-up with dialysis patients failed to reveal any further transmission.[1]

In total, Case D and his wife infected nine hospital staff members at this hospital and one patient. The facility was closed to new patients, and active surveillance for SARS was initiated.[1]

Phase Two

Toronto

After implementation of provincewide IPC measures in Canada, the number of recognized cases of SARS declined substantially, and no cases were detected after 20 April 2003.[6] On 30 April, the WHO lifted the travel advisory it had issued on 22 April that advised limiting travel to Toronto. Unfortunately, SARS was about to make a reappearance.

On 20 May 2003, several patients with SARS were discovered at a rehabilitation hospital in the north end of Toronto. The source of the infection was unclear; however, one of these cases was determined to have been hospitalized in the orthopedic ward of North York General Hospital between 22 and 28 April.[10,12]

The index case of this second Toronto outbreak was eventually determined to be a 96-year-old man who was admitted to North York General Hospital[12] on 22 March with a fractured pelvis. On 2 April, he was transferred to the orthopedic ward, where he had a fever and an infiltrate on a chest radiograph. Although he initially seemed to respond to antibiotics, on 19 April he again had respiratory symptoms, fever, and diarrhea. He had no apparent contact with anyone who had SARS, and an alternative diagnosis was determined for his problem. (In diagnosing SARS, if another diagnosis can be made, SARS is typically ruled out.) However, in subsequent investigation, several infected patients, visitors, and health care workers were all linked to this gentleman.[12]

On 23 May, North York General Hospital was closed to all new admissions other than patients with newly identified SARS. IPC practices were stepped up across several Toronto area hospitals. Staff at the hospital were placed on a 10-day work quarantine and instructed to avoid public places outside work, avoid contact with friends and family, and wear a mask whenever public contact was unavoidable.[12]

As a result of this second outbreak, SARS traveled to the United States via a North Carolina man who had visited a patient in a Toronto hospital. He was placed under quarantine at home with his family. Fortunately, the disease did not transmit any further.[13]

Hong Kong

Even before health and government officials knew exactly what they were facing, the spread of a new respiratory disease linked to China was a topic of great concern. Actions taken between February and June 2003, when the WHO removed Hong Kong from the list of areas with SARS outbreaks, included the following:[6]

- A surveillance system for cases of atypical pneumonia in public hospitals was established in response to reports of an epidemic in Guangdong Province, China.

- Private hospitals were asked to report cases of severe community-acquired pneumonia in response to reports of an epidemic in Guangdong Province, China.
- The Hong Kong Department of Health traced close contacts of patients presenting with symptoms.
- Hospitals closed wards with infected patients.
- Hong Kong added SARS to the list of infectious diseases in the Quarantine and Prevention of Diseases Ordinance.
- Medical centers were designated for surveillance of close contacts of infected patients.
- The Hospital Authority banned visitors in all acute wards.
- Close contacts of SARS patients were confined to their homes.

Implementing Control and Response Measures in Toronto

When organizations realized that SARS was not well controlled in Toronto, they began implementing several IPC and emergency management measures, including the following:

- Thorough and regular hand hygiene was practiced consistently.
- Gowns, hair and foot coverings, gloves, eye protection, and N95 or equivalent masks were provided for staff. Staff wore these N95 masks at all times while they were in the hospital.
- Single or negative pressure rooms were provided for all febrile patients.
- Dedicated equipment was provided for patients.
- Staff followed up with contacts of infected patients to monitor them for the disease.
- Patients were restricted to their rooms except for medically necessary tests.
- Staff were placed on quarantine at home with the exception of coming to work.
- Volunteers and medical students were excluded from the hospital.[2]
- Patients were not allowed visitors.
- Elective procedures, including those for some cancers, were postponed, and procedures that increased the risk of droplets were minimized.[4,11]
- Transfers between nursing homes and hospitals ceased.
- Hospitals sealed entrances and controlled access.[14]
- Health care workers minimized their contact with patients, including time spent in the patient's room.
- Hospitals introduced medical therapy to reduce coughing and vomiting.[4]

- Command centers were established in affected hospitals.
- The province of Ontario, in conjunction with nurses' and physicians' organizations, established a Provincial Operations Center for which all directives were given.
- Infectious disease experts were sent in from throughout Canada and the United States.[11]

An End to the Outbreaks in Hong Kong and Toronto

By mid-summer 2003, the SARS outbreak in Hong Kong and Canada appeared to be over. The illness had impacted six Hong Kong hospitals, two private clinics, and the large Amoy Gardens apartment complex. In the Toronto area, eight hospitals were hit with SARS. Psychologically and physically, these outbreaks affected thousands of patients, volunteers, and health care workers; harmed tourism; and caused other collateral damage that is still being felt today in both cities.

There is strong evidence that SARS was caused by a new form of coronavirus that was spread mainly via respiratory droplets and direct contact.[2] The incubation period for the disease ranged between 2 and 10 days, and although many tried, no one was able to create a reliable test for the disease. SARS, like other systemic respiratory diseases, remains a challenge to diagnose and manage because its early symptoms are indistinguishable from those of many other respiratory infections. Diagnosis is based on the clinical syndrome, a link to known cases of SARS, and the process of exclusion.[15] There is currently no vaccine for the disease, and experts are unsure about where, when, or if SARS will return.

Lessons Learned

Although the SARS outbreaks in Hong Kong and Toronto were difficult and often frightening experiences, some lessons can be learned from the outbreaks. Following is a discussion of some of those lessons.

Surveillance

Although collecting data to search for emerging infectious diseases has always been important, the SARS outbreak revealed glaring deficiencies in the world's surveillance system. By the time the WHO had released its alert and started active surveillance for SARS, the outbreak had already begun in Hong Kong and Toronto. The disease spread quickly, and surveillance systems in both countries were struggling to keep up.

One of the biggest risks of SARS is unrecognized patients.[4] If health care workers are unaware that a patient has SARS, they might not be as careful about using barrier precautions, allowing the disease to spread and infect more patients. Nowhere is this more clear than in Toronto's Phase Two outbreak. Because the health care workers at North York General Hospital were relaxing barrier precautions due to a slowdown in the outbreak, and because physicians made an inaccurate diagnosis, a patient was allowed to "slip through the cracks" and restart the SARS epidemic. Although some of the fallout was just incredibly bad luck, some experts have said that surveillance efforts during the crisis could certainly have been better.[4]

The keys to successful surveillance for emerging diseases involve comprehensive data collection, rapid detection of anomalies, early identification of issues, and rapid response. The tools for data collection and sharing must be consistent across local, regional, and national levels so that information can be compared and analyzed effectively. The use of technology to help surveillance efforts is an important step in developing an integrated surveillance system. Computers can sort through volumes of data quickly and reveal trends and patterns at the touch of a button. They also allow the communication and sharing of information electronically, which significantly speeds up the process of identification and response.

Laboratory support is also crucial to effective surveillance efforts. For example, local, regional, and national laboratories in Canada were responsible for testing patient specimens for SARS and reporting data to organizations across the country. Although Canada's laboratories engaged in a Herculean effort to rapidly test for SARS, some areas needed improvement. Standardized protocols and procedures for testing and communication could have been better, and resources for research were not sufficient. In anticipating an outbreak, laboratories should have policies and protocols that address some of the issues surrounding their participation in surveillance efforts, including the following:

- Specimen collection and transportation
- Biosafety measures for laboratory personnel
- Appropriate testing procedures
- Managing the volume of information that is present in an outbreak
- Timely presentation of testing and results
- Resource allotment for causal investigations and the development of diagnostic tests[16]
- Communication and collaboration between laboratories on an institutional, regional, and national level

Surveillance for emerging infectious disease should be multifaceted. Although laboratories, IPC professionals, and public health departments should all engage in comprehensive surveillance, staff of health care organizations must also bear some of the responsibility. Keeping a suspicious eye out for unusual presentations and unique symptoms can help rapidly identify the onset of an outbreak. If and when another SARS outbreak occurs, staff must remain vigilant and suspicious of unusual symptoms even as precautions are lessening and the epidemic appears over.

Communication

To say that it is important to communicate during a crisis such as SARS would be an understatement. Information and knowledge can help people make good decisions, identify issues, prevent panic, boost morale, and avoid adverse events. The only way that the large volume of individuals who needed information about SARS could all be well informed is through thorough, consistent, and effective communication. This involved information-sharing on two levels:

- Micro level—between leadership, physicians, nurses, laboratory personnel, IPC professionals, pharmacists, housekeeping staff, and engineering departments. By eliminating hierarchy, conducting briefings, and listening to each other, organizations can go a long way toward keeping staff motivated and in the loop.
- Macro level—between hospitals, with public health organizations, and between local governments and national entities. Using rapid communication strategies such as e-mail and faxing can help cut the time to share information across geographic areas.

Thinking about how and when individuals and organizations communicate with each other prior to an emergency can help facilitate effective communication when the time comes. Establishing a culture based on teamwork and flattened hierarchy while clearly identifying who is in charge during an emergency is critically important so that staff feel valued yet know that someone is looking out for their best interests. Predictability can be a comfort during an emergency, and establishing communication strategies prior to one can help ensure that communication is predictable under stress.

Effective communication can help to share knowledge, identify issues, and compare notes. SARS spread rapidly across multiple facilities in the greater Toronto area. By sharing information, the facilities could help control the spread of the disease, rapidly identify new cases, and share lessons learned as they came up. On the other hand, Hong Kong's early efforts to contain the outbreak likely were hampered by poor communication. The Department of Health learned of illness among health care staff at Prince of Wales Hospital only from the media. The lack of communication between the facility and public health officials shows how infectious outbreaks can appear to be contained without appropriate consideration of the potential effects on the community as a whole. Particularly during the early, confusing days of the rapid spread of an infection, ineffective communication can hamper early critical efforts to halt an outbreak. (*See* Sidebar 6-3 on page 155 for more details on health care system flaws revealed during the SARS outbreaks.)

Education

One of the more concerning aspects of Toronto's SARS outbreak was the infection of several health care workers who were using the appropriate

---

SIDEBAR 6-3

Exposing System Flaws

A government-sponsored investigation into the SARS epidemic in Hong Kong found a number of systems breakdowns in dealing with the outbreak at the Prince of Wales Hospital. Health care organizations planning for how they would respond to such a crisis at their facility can look to these identified issues to strengthen their efforts:

- Emergency management planning—an epidemic can quickly overwhelm contingency plans.
- Infection control planning—a comprehensive program for reducing the risk of health care–associated infections should include monitoring and clearly defined processes for reducing risk.
- Staff training—health care workers must understand how to spot infectious outbreaks and how to protect themselves and patients.
- Facility management—the design of patient care units, including ventilation and placement of beds, can be crucial in preventing the spread of infection.
- Equipment—necessary equipment to treat infected patients and properly protect against the spread of infection must be readily available.
- Communication—information about infections must be shared with external public health agencies.
- Partnerships—close collaboration between the public and private sectors is critical to identifying, treating, and containing infectious outbreaks.
- Surge capacity—organizations must plan for how they will handle an epidemic that severely strains resources such as staff, beds, supplies, and so forth.

---

barrier precautions. Although there is some debate about how they became infected, one of the considerations is that these staff members infected themselves when removing their protective equipment because they did not remove it in the optimal way. In Toronto, many health care workers lacked a clear understanding of the best ways to remove protective equipment without contaminating themselves.[17]

When under stress, individuals tend to rely on learned behaviors. Their memory is reduced, and their likelihood of correctly performing new procedures is affected. By thoroughly educating, training, and testing staff before an outbreak occurs, organizations can be sure that IPC measures are an automatic behavior that can be counted upon during high-stress situations. Following are some areas in which organizations should provide education and training:

- The proper use of barrier equipment, including gloves, gowns, eyewear, and masks
- The proper removal of barrier equipment to prevent the spread of infection

- Appropriate hand hygiene and use of gloves and other protective barriers, including the type, duration, and timing
- Optimal handling of infected patients
- Recognition of potential infectious diseases
- The role of staff in the emergency management plan, including knowing communication strategies and where to report

Organizations should be sure to include nonclinical staff in their training efforts. The housekeeping staff members who contracted SARS show that infectious diseases can effect all staff, not just those providing direct clinical care to the patients.

The Psychological Effects of a Biological Emergency

SARS did significantly more damage to the health care workers in Toronto and Hong Kong than causing morbidity and mortality. Those individuals who lived through the ordeal are still feeling the psychological and emotional effects. The uncertainty of whether they would get sick, the physical effects of wearing an N95 mask all the time, the emotional impact of not being able to touch family and friends, and the logistical and emotional hardships of being quarantined from everyone but their coworkers caused a tremendous strain on the health care profession in Toronto.

In retrospect, it is clear that some of these psychological scars could probably have been prevented or at least anticipated. An estimated 27,000 people were quarantined in the greater Toronto area over the course of the city's two outbreaks.[10] Hindsight is always perfect, and the international health community is now suggesting that such a comprehensive quarantine was probably not necessary. At the time, however, public health officials felt it was better to err on the side of caution.

Although it is hard to say whether quarantine decisions will be different the next time an unknown infectious disease appears, it is important that organizations anticipate the feelings of frustration, isolation, depression, fear, and helplessness that staff might feel as a result of such a quarantine. Nursing staff in particular felt the stress of the outbreak and quarantine because they were on rotating shifts and in many cases had the most contact with infected patients.

Every effort should be made to address the psychological and emotional needs of health care workers during an outbreak. Sometimes, just acknowledging the heroic work of health care professionals during a crisis can go a long way toward easing the pain associated with it. Other times, more tangible measures are necessary. Encouraging support groups and providing opportunities to talk with mental health professionals during the crisis can help. In addition, organizations might want to consider an insurance fund to cover health care workers who become sick or die through work.[18]

Staffing

As more people contracted SARS and more health care workers became sick, the staffing stresses upon health care organizations grew. SARS created a staffing nightmare for Toronto, which was already suffering from staff shortages.[14] ICUs and emergency departments were forced to close because of lack of staff, and, even in those areas that remained open, the provision of timely care was affected.

In many ways, the United States is fortunate that SARS didn't occur within its borders. One study by Kentucky researchers warns that the United States is ill-equipped for a SARS outbreak because of a shortage of epidemiologists, public-health nurses, and other staff.[19] It is important in preparing for the next infectious disease outbreak that organizations perform a comprehensive review of their staffing plans and make sure that they have or can get the appropriate number of professionals with the correct skill mix. Trying to staff a health care facility quickly is next to impossible, and preparation can go a long way toward ensuring effectiveness.

Limiting Collateral Damage

In addition to the obvious impact of SARS on Toronto and Hong Kong, the outbreaks caused the delay and cancellation of many types of health care procedures. Because of IPC risks and staffing limitations, for example, surgeries that under other circumstances would not have been considered elective suddenly were canceled or postponed in Toronto. The effect that these cancellations had on individuals is not easy to quantify, but one can assume they were significant. Organizations should consider this issue and work toward implementing plans that would allow for the continuation of other health care procedures during an outbreak so that the needs of the infected patients, as well as the needs of those who are not infected, are being met.

Although it is easy to look back and see what Hong Kong and Toronto could have done better, it is also easy to see that what happened in these two cities could happen anywhere. Health care organizations across the cities did an incredible job of limiting exposure, addressing issues, and stopping the spread of the disease. Organizations across the world would be wise to study the outbreaks and responses, and put plans in place that duplicate what was done right and address the areas where there were challenges.

References

1. Ontario SARS Scientific Advisory Committee, et al.: *Outbreak of SARS in Toronto, Ontario Phase 1: Tutor's Guide.* Teaching Module for Outbreaks. Aug. 2003. http://dante.med.utoronto.ca/doch/Year3/pdfs/TutorsSars.PDF (accessed Aug. 15, 2006).
2. Varia M., et al.: Investigation of a nosocomial outbreak of severe acute respiratory syndrome (SARS) in Toronto, Canada. *CMAJ* 169:285–292, Aug. 19, 2003.

3. Department of Health (Hong Kong): *Latest Figures on 2003 Severe Acute Respiratory Syndrome Outbreak (as of 19 January 2004).* 2004. www.info.gov.hk/dh/diseases/ap/eng/infected.htm (accessed Apr. 19, 2006).

4. McGeer A.: SARS in Toronto: Lessons for hospitals. Paper presented at the Joint Commission on Accreditation of Healthcare Organization's Infection Control Conference, Chicago, Nov. 17, 2003.

5. Tang P., et al.: Interpretation of diagnostic laboratory tests for severe acute respiratory syndrome: The Toronto experience. *CMAJ.* 170:47–54, Jan. 6, 2004.

6. SARS Expert Committee (Hong Kong): *SARS in Hong Kong: From Experience to Action, Summary Report, Chronology and Issues.* http://www.sars-expertcom.gov.hk/english/reports/summary/files/e_sumrpt_sect2.pdf (accessed Aug. 15, 2006).

7. Tsang K.W., et al.: A cluster of cases of severe acute respiratory syndrome in Hong Kong. *N Engl J Med* 348:1977–1985, May 2003.

8. Lee S.H.: The SARS epidemic in Hong Kong. *J Epidemiol Community Health* 57:652–654, Jun. 2003.

9. Hong Kong Health, Welfare and Food Bureau: *Health, Welfare and Food Bureau SARS Bulletin* Apr. 18, 2003. http://www.info.gov.hk/dh/diseases/ap/eng/bulletin0418.htm (accessed on Apr. 19, 2006).

10. Branswell H.: Big picture of SARS obscures tragedies. *Canadian Press,* Jul. 6, 2003. http://www.canada.com.

11. Update: Severe Acute Respiratory Syndrome—Toronto 2003. *MMWR Recomm Rep* 29, Jun. 13, 2003. http://www.cdc.gov/mmwr/preview/mmwrhtml/mm5223a4.htm (accessed Aug.15, 2006).

12. Associated Press: SARS in Toronto worrying World Health Organization. *Houston Chronicle,* Jun. 3, 2003. http://www.chron.com/cs/CDA/printstory.hts/special/sars/1935766 (accessed Oct. 18, 2005).

13. Associated Press: 12 patients show signs of SARS at Toronto hospital: Possible new cluster, link to NC case raise fears of another travel warning. *Baltimore Sun,* Jun. 11, 2003. http://www.newsday.com (accessed Oct. 18, 2005).

14. Caulford P.: SARS: Aftermath of an outbreak. *Lancet Extreme Medicine* 362, Dec. 2003. http://www.thelancet.com (Oct. 18, 2005).

15. National Advisory Committee on SARS and Public Health: *Learning from SARS. A Report of the National Advisory Committee on SARS and Public Health.* Ottawa, ON; Health Canada, Oct. 2003.

16. Health Canada: *Health Canada's Preparedness for and Response to Respiratory Infections Season and the Possible Re-emergence of SARS.* Nov. 19, 2003. http://www.phac-aspc.gc.ca/sars-sras/ris-sir/index.html (accessed Aug. 15, 2006).

17. Centers for Disease Control and Prevention: Cluster of severe acute respiratory syndrome cases among protected healthcare workers: Toronto, Canada, Apr. 2003. *Morb Mortal Wkly Rpt* 52:433–436, May 16, 2003.

18. Singer P., et al.: Ethics and SARS: Lessons from Toronto. *BMJ* 327:1342–1344, Dec. 6, 2003.

19. New outbreak could devastate poor countries, Canadian intelligence agency says. *TB & Outbreaks Week* p. 48, Dec. 30, 2003.

Resources

The following readings were gathered for use in *Information Resources in Infection Control,* Fourth Edition (Editor: Nizam Damani M.D., MBBS, MSc, FRCPI, FRCPath), due in 2006 from the International Federation of Infection Control (IFIC). The full document will be available online at IFIC's Web site: http://www.theific.org/publications.asp. NOTE: Some of these resources may appear at the end of more than one chapter, due to their applicability to more than one aspect of infection prevention and control.

Association for Professionals in Infection Control and Epidemiology, Inc./Community and Hospital Infection Control Association-Canada: Professional and practice standards. *Am J Infect Control* 27:1; 47–51, 1999.

Centers for Disease Control and Prevention: *SARS Preparedness in Healthcare Facilities.* May 3, 2005. http://www.cdc.gov/ncidod/sars/guidance/C/app2.htm.

Health Protection Agency: *SARS: Hospital Infection Control Guidance.* Nov. 2005. http://www.hpa.org.uk/infections/topics_az/SARS/ hosp_infect_cont.htm.

Public Health Agency of Canada: *Severe Respiratory Illness (SRI) in the SARS "Post-Outbreak" Period.* Jan. 2005. http://www.phac-aspc.gc.ca/ sars-sras/prof_e.html.

World Health Organization: *Alert, Verification and Public Health Management of SARS in the Post-Outbreak Period.* Aug. 14, 2003. http://www.who.int/csr/ sars/postoutbreak/en.

———: *Hospital Infection Control Guidance for Severe Acute Respiratory Syndrome (SARS).* 2003. http://www.who.int/csr/sars/infectioncontrol/en/.

———: *Interim Guidelines for National SARS Preparedness.* Manila: Regional Office for Western Pacific, WHO, 2003.

World Health Organization: *Guidelines on prevention and control of hospital associated infections.* New Delhi: WHO Regional Office for South East Asia, 2002. Document no. SEA-HLM-343.

JCI Prevention and Control of Infections Standards and Compliance Checklist

Use the checklist on the following pages to assess compliance with JCI's Prevention and Control of Infections (PCI) standards, as described in Chapter 2 of this book. Each checklist box assesses compliance with the measurable elements (ME) of each standard. Please note that these standards are effective as of the date of this publication (October 2006), but hospital standards will be updated in 2007.

Standard PCI.1	**Standard Score:** ❏ Compliant		❏ Not Compliant	
Assessment Questions	**Level of Compliance**	**Evidence of Compliance**	**Plan of Action**	**Due Date**
1. Does a program exist to reduce the risk of nosocomial infections in patients and health care workers?				
2. Is the program appropriate to the organization's size and geographic location, services, and patients?				

Standard PCI.1.1	**Standard Score:** ❏ Compliant		❏ Not Compliant	
Assessment Question	**Level of Compliance**	**Evidence of Compliance**	**Plan of Action**	**Due Date**
1. Are all areas of the organization included in the infection prevention and control program?				

Standard PCI.2	**Standard Score:** ❏ Compliant		❏ Not Compliant	
Assessment Questions	**Level of Compliance**	**Evidence of Compliance**	**Plan of Action**	**Due Date**
1. Has the organization established the focus of the program to prevent or reduce the incidence of nosocomial infections?				
2. Are respiratory tract infections included as appropriate to the organization?				
3. Are urinary tract infections included as appropriate to the organization?				
4. Are intravascular invasive devices included as appropriate to the organization?				
5. Are surgical wounds included as appropriate to the organization?				

Standard PCI.3	Standard Score: ❑ Compliant		❑ Not Compliant	
Assessment Questions	**Level of Compliance**	**Evidence of Compliance**	**Plan of Action**	**Due Date**
1. Has the organization identified those processes associated with infection risk and implemented strategies to reduce infection risk in those processes?				
2. Are equipment cleaning and sterilization included as appropriate to the organization?				
3. Is laundry and linen management included as appropriate to the organization?				
4. Is disposal of infectious waste and body fluids included as appropriate to the organization?				
5. Is the handling and disposal of blood and blood components included as appropriate to the organization?				
6. Are kitchen sanitation and food preparation and handling included as appropriate to the organization?				
7. Is the operation of the mortuary and postmortem area included as appropriate to the organization?				
8. Is the disposal of sharps and needles included as appropriate to the organization?				
9. Is separation of patients with communicable diseases from patients and staff who are at greater risk due to immunosuppression or other reasons included as appropriate to the organization?				
10. Is the management of hemorrhagic (bleeding) patients included as appropriate to the organization?				
11. Are engineering controls included as appropriate to the organization?				

Standard PCI.4	Standard Score: ❑ Compliant		❑ Not Compliant	
Assessment Questions	**Level of Compliance**	**Evidence of Compliance**	**Plan of Action**	**Due Date**
1. Does the organization identify those situations for which gloves and masks are required?				
2. Are gloves and masks correctly used in those situations?				
3. Does the organization identify those areas where hand-washing and disinfecting procedures are required?				
4. Are hand-washing and disinfecting procedures used correctly in those areas?				

Standard PCI.5	Standard Score: ❑ Compliant		❑ Not Compliant	
Assessment Questions	**Level of Compliance**	**Evidence of Compliance**	**Plan of Action**	**Due Date**
1. Does the organization identify those sites from which specimens are to be collected and the frequency of the collection from each site?				
2. Are specimens routinely collected?				
3. Are specimens collected and handled properly?				

Standard PCI.6	Standard Score: ❑ Compliant		❑ Not Compliant	
Assessment Questions	**Level of Compliance**	**Evidence of Compliance**	**Plan of Action**	**Due Date**
1. Do one or more individuals oversee the infection prevention and control program?				
2. Are the individuals qualified for the scope and complexity of the program?				

Standard PCI.7	**Standard Score:** ❑ Compliant		❑ Not Compliant	
Assessment Question	**Level of Compliance**	**Evidence of Compliance**	**Plan of Action**	**Due Date**
1. Is responsibility for coordinating the overall program assigned to one individual, a committee, or other mechanism?				

Standard PCI.8	**Standard Score:** ❑ Compliant		❑ Not Compliant	
Assessment Questions	**Level of Compliance**	**Evidence of Compliance**	**Plan of Action**	**Due Date**
1. Do coordination of infection prevention and control activities involve medicine?				
2. Do coordination of infection prevention and control activities involve nursing?				
3. Do coordination of infection prevention and control activities involve others as appropriate to the organization?				

Standard PCI.9	**Standard Score:** ❑ Compliant		❑ Not Compliant	
Assessment Questions	**Level of Compliance**	**Evidence of Compliance**	**Plan of Action**	**Due Date**
1. Is the infection prevention and control program based on current scientific knowledge?				
2. Is the infection prevention and control program based on accepted practice guidelines?				
3. Is the infection prevention and control program based on applicable law and regulation?				

Standard PCI.10	**Standard Score:** ❑ Compliant		❑ Not Compliant	
Assessment Question	**Level of Compliance**	**Evidence of Compliance**	**Plan of Action**	**Due Date**
1. Do information management systems support the infection prevention and control program?				

Standard PCI.11	**Standard Score:** ❑ Compliant		❑ Not Compliant	
Assessment Question	**Level of Compliance**	**Evidence of Compliance**	**Plan of Action**	**Due Date**
1. Are infection prevention and control activities integrated into the organization's quality improvement and patient safety program?				

Standard PCI.11.1	**Standard Score:** ❑ Compliant		❑ Not Compliant	
Assessment Questions	**Level of Compliance**	**Evidence of Compliance**	**Plan of Action**	**Due Date**
1. Are nosocomial infection risks tracked?				
2. Are nosocomial infection rates tracked?				
3. Are nosocomial infection trends tracked?				

Standard PCI.11.2	**Standard Score:** ❑ Compliant		❑ Not Compliant	
Assessment Questions	**Level of Compliance**	**Evidence of Compliance**	**Plan of Action**	**Due Date**
1. Does infection monitoring use indicator measures?				
2. Do the indicators measure epidemiologically important infections?				

Standard PCI.11.3	Standard Score: ❑ Compliant		❑ Not Compliant	
Assessment Questions	**Level of Compliance**	**Evidence of Compliance**	**Plan of Action**	**Due Date**
1. Are processes redesigned based on risk, rate, and trend data and information?				
2. Are processes redesigned to reduce infection risk to the lowest levels possible?				

Standard PCI.11.4	Standard Score: ❑ Compliant		❑ Not Compliant	
Assessment Question	**Level of Compliance**	**Evidence of Compliance**	**Plan of Action**	**Due Date**
1. Are infection prevention and control rates compared to other organizations' rates?				

Standard PCI.11.5	Standard Score: ❑ Compliant		❑ Not Compliant	
Assessment Questions	**Level of Compliance**	**Evidence of Compliance**	**Plan of Action**	**Due Date**
1. Are monitoring results communicated to medical staff?				
2. Are monitoring results communicated to nursing staff?				
3. Are monitoring results communicated to management?				

Standard PCI.11.6	Standard Score: ❑ Compliant		❑ Not Compliant	
Assessment Question	**Level of Compliance**	**Evidence of Compliance**	**Plan of Action**	**Due Date**
1. Are infection prevention and control program results reported to public health agencies as required?				

Standard PCI.12	**Standard Score:** ❏ Compliant		❏ Not Compliant	
Assessment Questions	**Level of Compliance**	**Evidence of Compliance**	**Plan of Action**	**Due Date**
1. Does the organization provide education about infection prevention and control?				
2. Are medical, nursing, and other professional staff included in the program?				
3. Are patients and families included when appropriate to the patient's needs and condition?				

Standard PCI.12.1	**Standard Score:** ❏ Compliant		❏ Not Compliant	
Assessment Question	**Level of Compliance**	**Evidence of Compliance**	**Plan of Action**	**Due Date**
1. Are staff oriented to the policies, procedures, and practices of the infection prevention and control program?				

Standard PCI.12.2	**Standard Score:** ❏ Compliant		❏ Not Compliant	
Assessment Questions	**Level of Compliance**	**Evidence of Compliance**	**Plan of Action**	**Due Date**
1. Does periodic staff education include new policies and procedures?				
2. Is periodic staff education provided in response to significant trends in infection data?				

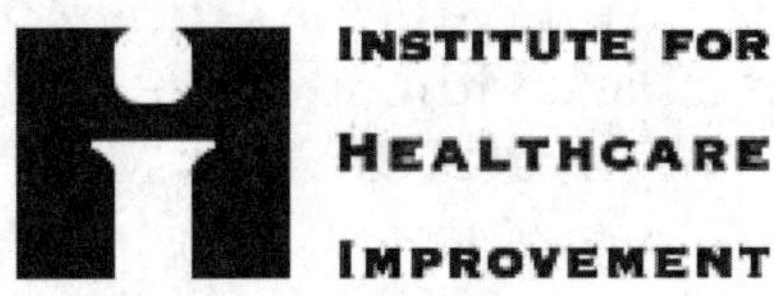

How-to Guide:
Improving Hand Hygiene

A Guide for Improving Practices
among Health Care Workers

This guide was prepared in collaboration with the Centers for Disease Control and Prevention (CDC), the Association for Professionals in Infection Control and Epidemiology (APIC), and the Society of Healthcare Epidemiology of America (SHEA), and has been endorsed by APIC and SHEA. Valuable input also was provided by the World Health Organization's World Alliance for Patient Safety through the Global Patient Safety Challenge.

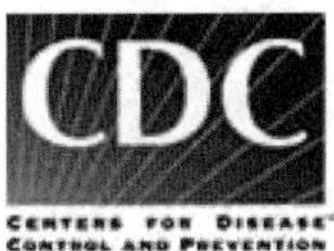

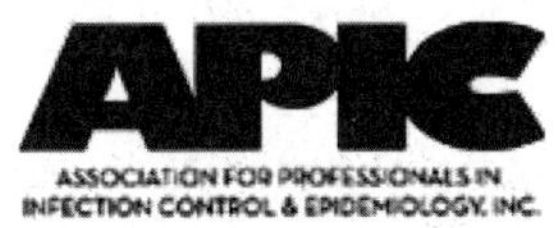

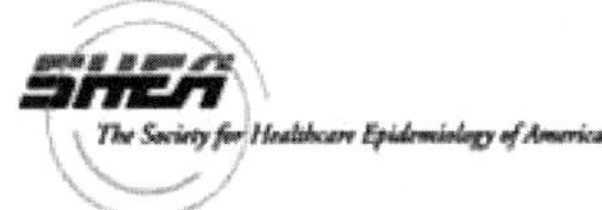

Acknowledgments

The Institute for Healthcare Improvement (IHI) acknowledges the valuable contributions of the following individuals:

- W. Charles Huskins, MD, MSc; Assistant Professor of Pediatrics, Mayo Clinic College of Medicine, Consultant, Pediatric Infectious Diseases, Mayo Clinic, Rochester, MN
- John M. Boyce, MD; Chief, Infectious Diseases Section, Hospital of Saint Raphael, New Haven, CT (SHEA)
- Loretta Litz Fauerbach, MS, CIC; Director, Infection Control, Shands Hospital at the University of Florida, Gainesville, FL (APIC)
- Barbara I. Braun, PhD; Project Director, Center for Health Services Research, Division of Research, JCAHO
- Nancy Kupka, DNSc, MPH, RN; Project Director, Division of Standards and Survey Methods, JCAHO
- Linda Kusek, Rn, BSN, MPH; Associate Project Director, Division of Research, JCAHO

The purpose of this guide is to help organizations reduce health-care-associated infections, including infections due to antibiotic-resistant organisms, by improving hand hygiene practices and use of gloves among health care workers.

The Case for Improving Hand Hygiene and Use of Gloves among Health Care Workers

Health-care-associated infections are an important cause of morbidity and mortality among hospitalized patients worldwide. Such infections affect nearly 2 million individuals annually in the United States and are responsible for approximately 80,000 deaths each year. Transmission of health-care-associated pathogens most often occurs via the contaminated hands of health care workers. Accordingly, hand hygiene (i.e., handwashing with soap and water or use of a waterless, alcohol-based hand rub) has long been considered one of the most important infection control measures for preventing health-care-associated infections. However, compliance by health care workers with recommended hand hygiene procedures has remained unacceptable, with compliance rates generally below 50% of hand hygiene opportunities.

> ➤ Jarvis WR. Selected aspects of the socioeconomic impact of nosocomial infections: Morbidity, mortality, cost, and prevention. *Infect Control Hosp Epidemiol.* 1996 Aug;17(8):552-557.

> ➤ Pittet D, Mourouga P, Perneger TV. Compliance with handwashing in a teaching hospital. *Ann Intern Med.* 1999;130:126-130.

> ➤ Lankford MG, Zemblower TR, Trick WE, Hacek DM, Noskin GA, Peterson LR. Influence of role models and hospital design on hand hygiene of healthcare workers. *Emerg Infect Dis.* 2003;9:217-23.

Many factors have contributed to poor handwashing compliance among health care workers, including a lack of knowledge among personnel about the importance of hand hygiene in reducing the spread of infection and how hands become contaminated, lack of understanding of correct hand hygiene technique, understaffing and overcrowding, poor access to handwashing facilities, irritant contact dermatitis associated with frequent exposure to soap and water, and lack of institutional commitment to good hand hygiene.

> ➤ Pittet D, Boyce JM. Hand hygiene and patient care: Pursuing the Semmelweis legacy. *Lancet Infect Dis.* 2001;1:9-20.

To overcome these barriers, the Centers for Disease Control and Prevention's (CDC's) Healthcare Infection Control Practices Advisory Committee (HICPAC) published a comprehensive *Guideline for Hand Hygiene in Health-Care Settings* in 2002. One of the principal recommendations of this guideline was that waterless, alcohol-based hand rubs (liquids, gels or foams) are the preferred method for hand hygiene in most situations due to the superior efficacy of these agents in rapidly reducing bacterial counts on hands and their ease of use. Alcohol preparations also rapidly kill many fungi and viruses that cause health-care-associated infections. The guideline recommended that health care facilities develop multidimensional programs to improve hand hygiene practices.

➤ Boyce JM, Pittet D, et al. Guideline for Hand Hygiene in Health-Care Settings: Recommendations of the Healthcare Infection Control Practices Advisory Committee and the HICPAC/SHEA/APIC/IDSA Hand Hygiene Task Force. *Morbid Mortal Wkly Rep.* 2002;51(RR16):1-45.

Recognizing a worldwide need to improve hand hygiene in health care facilities, the World Health Organization (WHO) launched its *Guidelines on Hand Hygiene in Health Care (Advanced Draft)* in October 2005. These global consensus guidelines reinforce the need for multidimensional strategies as the most effective approach to promote hand hygiene. Key elements include staff education and motivation, adoption of an alcohol-based hand rub as the primary method for hand hygiene, use of performance indicators, and strong commitment by all stakeholders, such as front-line staff, managers and health care leaders, to improve hand hygiene.

➤ *WHO Guidelines on Hand Hygiene in Health Care (Advanced Draft): A Summary.* World Health Organization; 2005. [Available online at http://www.who.int/patientsafety/events/05/HH_en.pdf]

Wearing gloves during patient care is an additional intervention to help reduce transmission of infectious agents in high-risk situations. Gloves protect patients by reducing contamination of the health care worker's hands and subsequent transmission of pathogens to other patients. In addition, when gloves are worn in compliance with CDC's Standard Precautions, gloves protect health care workers from exposure to bloodborne infections such as HIV and hepatitis B and C.

However, gloves must be used properly. Gloves can become contaminated during care and must be removed or changed when moving from a contaminated site to a clean site on the same patient. Gloved hands can also become contaminated due to tiny punctures in the glove material or during glove removal; therefore, hand hygiene must be performed immediately after glove removal. Consequently, use of gloves is an important adjunct to, but not a replacement for, proper hand hygiene practice.

➤ Pittet D, et al. Bacterial contamination of the hands of hospital Staff during routine patient care. *Arch Intern Med.* 1999;159:821-826.

➤ Pessoa-Silva CL, Richtmann R, Calil et al. Dynamics of bacterial hand contamination during routine neonatal care. *Infect Control and Hosp Epidemiol.* 2004;25:192-197.

➤ Tenorio AR, Badri SM, Sahgal NB, et al. Effectiveness of gloves in the prevention of hand carriage of vancomycin-resistant Enterococcus species by health care workers after patient care. *Clin Infect Dis.* 2001;32:826–829.

➤ Johnson S, Gerding DN, et al. Prospective, controlled study of vinyl glove use to interrupt Clostridium difficile nosocomial transmission. *Am J Med.* 1990;88:137-140.

> Garner JS, Hospital Infection Control Practices Advisory Committee. Guideline for isolation precautions in hospitals. *Infect Control Hosp Epidemiol.* 1996;17:53-80. [Available online at http://www.cdc.gov/ncidod/dhqp/gl_isolation.html]

The Potential Impact of Improving Hand Hygiene

Numerous studies have suggested that hand hygiene compliance can be improved, at least modestly, by a variety of interventions, introduction of alcohol-based hand rub and educational and behavioral initiatives. Most authorities believe that multidimensional interventions are more effective. For example, Pittet et al. implemented a multidisciplinary, multimodal hand hygiene improvement program featuring promotion of alcohol-based hand rub and achieved substantial improvement in hand hygiene compliance. Much of the improvement in compliance was attributed to increased use of the alcohol-based hand rub. As hand hygiene compliance improved, both the incidence of nosocomial infections and new methicillin-resistant *Staphylococcus aureus* (MRSA) cases decreased, although the authors did not assert that they had rigorously demonstrated a causal link (see figures below).

> Pittet D, Hugonnet S, et al. Effectiveness of a hospital-wide programme to improve compliance with hand hygiene. *Lancet.* 2000;356:1307-1312.

The Hand Hygiene Intervention Package

The hand hygiene intervention package is a group of best practices that individually improve care, but when applied together should result in substantially greater improvement. The science supporting each intervention is sufficiently established to be considered a standard of care.

The following four components of the hand hygiene intervention package are critical aspects of a multidimensional hand hygiene program. Glove use is included in this package because proper glove use is inextricably linked to effective hand hygiene.

1. Clinical staff, including new hires and trainees, understand key elements of hand hygiene practice (demonstrate knowledge)
2. Clinical staff, including new hires and trainees, use appropriate technique when cleansing their hands (demonstrate competence)
3. Alcohol-based hand rub and gloves are available at the point of care (enable staff)
4. Hand hygiene is performed at the right time and in the right way and gloves are used appropriately as recommended by CDC's Standard Precautions (verify competency, monitor compliance, and provide feedback)

1. Clinical staff, including new hires and trainees, understand key elements of hand hygiene practice (demonstrate knowledge)

Health care workers' hands can become contaminated by touching the body secretions, excretions, nonintact skin, and wounds of patients; however, they can also

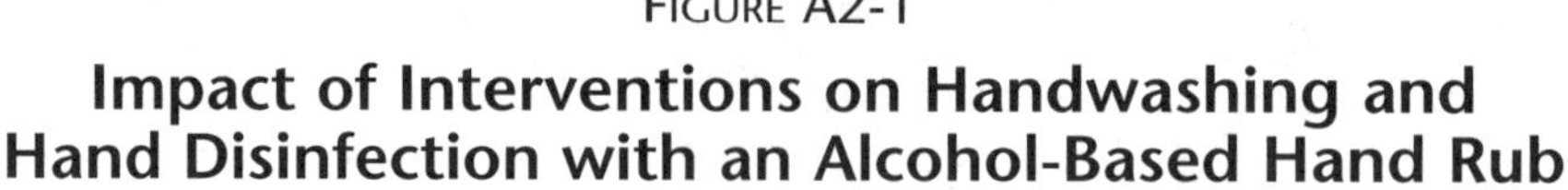

Impact of Interventions on Handwashing and Hand Disinfection with an Alcohol-Based Hand Rub

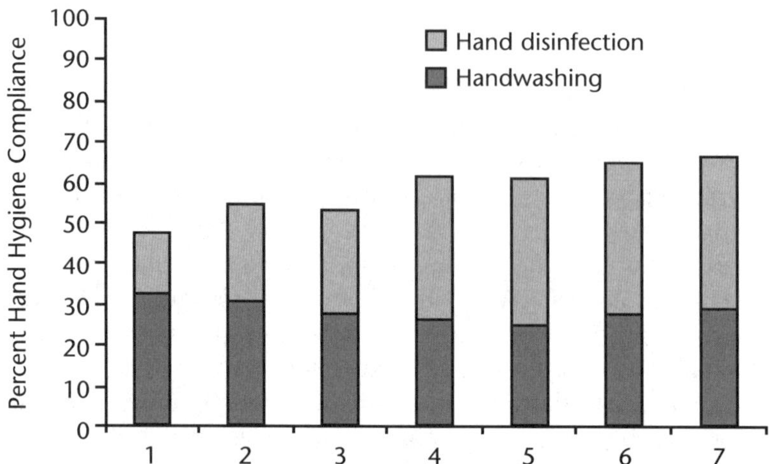

Figure A2-2

Impact of Hand Hygiene on Incidence of Methicillin-Resistant *Staphylcoccus aureus* (MRSA) and Nosocomial Infections

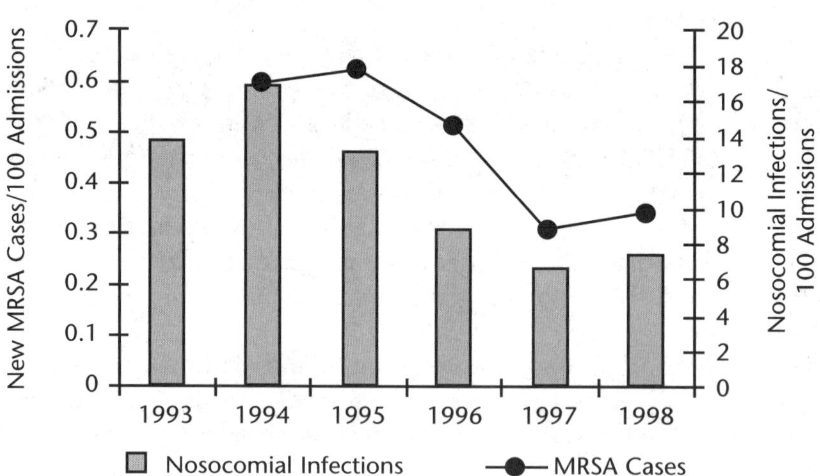

become contaminated by touching intact skin of patients and environmental surfaces in the immediate vicinity of the patients. Health care workers should demonstrate accurate knowledge that their hands can become contaminated during all of these activities.

> Pittet D, Dharan S, Touveneau S, Savan V, Perneger TVI. Bacterial contamination of the hands of hospital staff during routine patient care. *Arch Intern Med.* 1999;159:821-826. ¾ Duckro AN, Blom DW, Lyle EA, Weinstein RA, Hayden MKI. Transfer of vancomycin-resistant enterococci via health care worker hands. *Arch Intern Med.* 2005;165:302-307.

Compared to handwashing, alcohol-based hand rubs have been shown to be more effective in reducing the number of viable bacteria and viruses on hands, require less time to use, can be made more accessible at the point of care, and cause less hand irritation and dryness with repeated use. Handwashing is required when hands are visibly contaminated and is also appropriate after caring for patients with diarrhea, including patients with *Clostridium difficile* associated diarrhea, before eating, and after use of the restroom. Health care workers should demonstrate accurate knowledge of the advantages of the use of hand rubs in most situations as well as the specific indications for handwashing.

> Boyce JM, Pittet D. Guideline for Hand Hygiene in Health-Care Settings: Recommendations of the Healthcare Infection Control Practices Advisory Committee and the HICPAC/SHEA/APIC/IDSA Hand Hygiene Task Force. *Morbid Mortal Wkly Rep.* 2002;51:1-45.

> *WHO Guidelines on Hand Hygiene in Health Care (Advanced Draft): A Summary.* World Health Organization; 2005. [Available online at http://www.who.int/patientsafety/events/05/HH_en.pdf]

What changes can we make that will result in improvement?

Hospital teams across the United States and in other countries around the world have developed and tested change strategies that allowed them to improve knowledge of key elements of hand hygiene practice. Successful strategies include:

* Discussing the types of patient care activities that result in hand contamination as a supplement to educational material provided to health care workers
* Discussing with clinical staff the relative advantages and disadvantages of handwashing and use of alcohol-based hand rubs at the point of care
* Emphasizing the important role that contaminated hands play in transmission of health-care-associated pathogens, including multidrug-resistant pathogens and viruses
* Informing clinical staff of the morbidity and mortality caused by health-care-associated infections

2. Clinical staff, including new hires and trainees, use appropriate technique when cleansing their hands (demonstrate competency)

To be optimally effective, an appropriate volume of alcohol-based hand rub or soap must be applied to all surfaces of the hands and fingers for a sufficient length of time. Failure to do so will reduce the efficacy of the hand hygiene regimen. Accordingly, clinical staff should demonstrate competency in performing hand hygiene correctly. Competent hand rubbing requires that a sufficient volume of an alcohol-based rub is applied to cover all surfaces of the hands and fingers and that at least 15 seconds of rubbing is necessary before the hands are dry. Competent handwashing requires that a sufficient volume of soap is applied to cover all surfaces of the hands and fingers, and that at least 15 seconds of scrubbing with friction is performed before rinsing. Care should be taken to avoid contamination of hands after handwashing (paper towels or single use cloth towels should be used; if the faucet is hand-operated, the towel should be used to turn of the spigot).

> Larson EL, Eke PI, Wilder MP, Laughon BE. Quantity of soap as a variable in handwashing. *Infect Control.* 1987;8:371–375.

> Widmer AE, Dangel M. Alcohol-based hand rub: Evaluation of technique and microbiological efficacy with international infection control professionals. *Infect Control Hosp Epidemiol.* 2004;25:207–209.

What changes can we make that will result in improvement?

Hospital teams have developed and tested change strategies that allow them to improve competence with hand hygiene practices. Some of these changes include:

- Conducting live demonstrations of correct techniques for using an alcohol-based hand rub and handwashing during educational sessions for health care workers
- Providing videotape presentations of correct handwashing and hand rubbing technique in educational material for health care workers
- Emphasizing that an appropriate volume of hand rub or soap must be used if hand hygiene is to be effective
- Using fluorescent dye-based training methods to demonstrate correct hand hygiene techniques to clinical staff
- Periodically monitoring the adequacy of hand hygiene technique among clinical staff, and giving them feedback regarding their performance

3. Alcohol-based hand rub and gloves are available at the point of care (enable staff)

Placing alcohol-based hand rub dispensers near the point of care has been associated with increased compliance by health care workers with recommended hand hygiene procedures.

For example, Bischoff et al. found that compliance by health care workers was significantly greater when dispensers for alcohol-based hand rub were adjacent to each patient's bed than when there was only one dispenser for every four beds. In critical care, availability of alcohol-based hand rub at the point of care proved to minimize the time constraint associated with hand hygiene during patient care and to predict better compliance. In a study of hand hygiene among physicians, Pittet et al. found that easy access to an alcohol-based hand rub was an independent predictor of improved hand hygiene compliance.

> Bischoff WE, Reynolds TM, Sessler CN, Edmond MB, Wenzel RP. Handwashing compliance by health care workers: The impact of introducing an accessible, alcohol-based hand antiseptic. *Arch Intern Med.* 2000;160:1017–1021.

> Pittet D, Hugonnet S, et al. Effectiveness of a hospital-wide programme to improve compliance with hand hygiene. *Lancet.* 2000;356:1307-1312.

> Hugonnet S, Perneger TV, Pittet D. Alcohol-based hand rub improves compliance with hand hygiene in intensive care units. *Arch Int Med.* 2002;162:1037–1043.

> Pittet D, Simon A, Hugonnet S, et al. Hand hygiene among physicians: Performance, beliefs, and perceptions. *Ann Intern Med.* 2004;148:1-8.

Availability of alcohol-based products at the point of care should be supplemented by availability of gloves in appropriate sizes for use in the high-risk situations described previously for which barrier technique is indicated. Sterile gloves are not required for this purpose; studies have shown that clean single-use gloves have negligible numbers of non-pathogenic microorganisms when cultured.

What changes can we make that will result in improvement?

Hospital teams that have developed and tested change strategies to make alcohol-based hand rub and clean gloves readily available to health care workers saw improved hand hygiene compliance. Some of these changes include:
- Placing dispensers for alcohol-based hand rub and boxes of clean gloves of various sizes near the point of care, such as:
  - Next to each patient's bed
  - Attached to the frame of patient beds
  - Near the door to each patient's room (either adjacent to the door in the corridor or just inside the door)
  - At nursing stations or on medication carts
  - Supplied as portable (pocket or belt) individual dispensers for personal use
- Installing alcohol-based hand rub dispensers in locations that are compliant with local and federal fire safety regulations
- Assigning responsibility for checking alcohol-based hand rub dispensers and glove boxes on a regular basis to assure that:
  - Dispensers and glove boxes are not empty
  - Dispensers are operational
  - Dispensers provide the correct amount of the product

- Evaluating the design and function of dispensers before selecting a product for use since poorly functioning dispensers may adversely affect hand hygiene compliance rates

4. Hand hygiene is performed and gloves are used appropriately as recommended by CDC's Standard Precautions (verify competency, monitor compliance, and provide feedback)

Clinical staff should clean their hands according to recommendations listed in the CDC *Guideline for Hand Hygiene in Health-Care Settings*. These recommendations include:

- Washing hands with plain soap or with antimicrobial soap and water, as follows:
  - When hands are visibly dirty or contaminated with proteinaceous material or with blood or other body fluids
  - Before eating
  - After using the restroom
  - After caring for patients colonized with *Clostridium difficile*
- If hands are not visibly soiled, use an alcohol-based hand rub for routinely decontaminating hands in the following situations:
  - Before direct contact with patients
  - Before donning sterile gloves when inserting a central intravascular catheter
  - Before inserting indwelling urinary catheters, peripheral vascular catheters, or other invasive devices
  - After direct contact with a patient's skin
  - After contact with body fluids, mucous membranes, nonintact skin, and wound dressings if hands are not visibly soiled
  - When moving from a contaminated body site to a clean body site during patient care
  - After contact with inanimate objects in the immediate vicinity of the patient
  - After removing gloves
- If there has been any contact with the patient or the patient's environment, hands should be decontaminated when leaving the patient's bedside or room

➤ Boyce JM, Pittet D, et al. Guideline for Hand Hygiene in Health-Care Settings: Recommendations of the Healthcare Infection Control Practices Advisory Committee and the HICPAC/SHEA/APIC/IDSA Hand Hygiene Task Force. *Morbid Mortal Wkly Rep.* 2002;51(RR16):1-45.

➤ *WHO Guidelines on Hand Hygiene in Health Care (Advanced Draft): A Summary.* World Health Organization; 2005. [Available online at http://www.who.int/patientsafety/events/05/HH_en.pdf]

Clinical staff should wear gloves according to recommendations listed in CDC's Standard Precautions. These recommendations include:

- Wearing gloves when contact with blood or other potentially infectious body fluids, excretions, secretions (except sweat), mucous membranes, and nonintact skin could occur
- Removing gloves after caring for a patient—personnel should not wear the same pair of gloves for the care of more than one patient
- Changing gloves during patient care when moving from a contaminated body site to a clean body site
- Performing hand hygiene immediately after removal of gloves

➤ Garner JS, Hospital Infection Control Practices Advisory Committee. Guideline for isolation precautions in hospitals. *Infect Control Hosp Epidemiol.* 1996;17:53-80. [Available online at http://www.cdc.gov/ncidod/dhqp/gl_isolation.html]

➤ *WHO Guidelines on Hand Hygiene in Health Care (Advanced Draft): A Summary.* World Health Organization; 2005. [Available online at http://www.who.int/patientsafety/events/05/HH_en.pdf]

What changes can we make that will result in improvement?

Hospital teams have developed and tested change strategies that allow them to improve hand hygiene practice and use of gloves by health care workers. Some of these changes include:

- Incorporating the indications for hand hygiene and use of gloves in educational material presented to health care workers. Examples of educational materials include:
  - Periodic lectures given by knowledgeable personnel, including interactive, audience-response software, if possible
  - Videotapes and PowerPoint presentations that demonstrate the importance of proper hand hygiene techniques in health care settings
  - Interactive, computer-assisted learning available to clinical staff via the hospital's Intranet
- Conducting educational programs for personnel that include instructions for proper technique when washing hands with soap and water, or when using an alcohol-based hand rub
- Ensuring that providers understand the rationale for hand hygiene and gloves and can comply with best practices and improve patient outcomes (self-efficacy)
- Initiating a multi-component publicity campaign (e.g., posters with photos of celebrated hospital doctors/staff members recommending hand hygiene and use of gloves; drawings by children in pediatric hospitals; screen savers with targeted messaging)
- Using opinion leaders as role models and educators ("academic detailing")

- Creating a culture where reminding each other about hand hygiene and use of gloves is encouraged and makes compliance the social norm
- Enabling health care workers to comply with best hand hygiene and glove practices by creating reliable systems that ensure alcohol-based hand hygiene products and gloves in appropriate sizes are always readily available at the point of care
- Engage patients and families in hand hygiene efforts by providing patient safety "tip sheets" outlining appropriate hand hygiene and glove practices, and encouraging them to remind health care providers to comply with these standards
- Monitoring compliance by health care workers with recommended indications for hand hygiene and use of gloves, including real-time feedback to personnel and trending compliance over time

How to Begin Improvement in Your Organization

Forming the Team

The Institute for Healthcare Improvement (IHI) recommends a multidisciplinary team approach to improving hand hygiene among health care workers. Improvement teams should be heterogeneous in make-up, but unified in mindset. The value of bringing diverse personnel together is that all members of the care team are given a stake in the outcome and work together to achieve the same goal.

Including all stakeholders in the process to implement proper hand hygiene techniques will help gain buy-in and cooperation of all parties. For example, teams without nurses are bound to fail. Teams led by nurses and therapists may be successful, but often lack leverage; physicians must also be part of the team. The team should include, at a minimum, an administrator or senior leader who can help remove barriers to implementation, as well as a member of the department that supplies hand hygiene agents to clinical areas. Involve the team in designing or selecting hand hygiene posters or other motivational and educational materials.

Some suggestions for attracting and retaining excellent team members include: using data to define and solve the problem; finding champions and opinion leaders within the hospital to lend the effort immediate credibility; and engaging individuals who want to work on the project rather than trying to convince those who do not.

Commitment of institutional leadership is a key determinant of success. There must be alignment of leadership, including the board, executives, heads of clinical departments, and the infection control team. Leadership should give encouragement, set expectations, remove barriers, and celebrate success. Concrete, "raise-the-bar" goals (i.e., those that strive to achieve unprecedented levels of performance) set the stage for achieving rates of compliance well beyond historical levels. An "all-or-none" mentality for compliance (i.e., performing all elements of good practice) is necessary to achieve the highest possible levels of reliable performance. From the patient's perspective, compliance with all elements of appropriate hand hygiene and glove practice is a reasonable expectation.

Once high levels of compliance are achieved, a "process owner" must be identified—the person who will ensure that high levels of performance are maintained and help to troubleshoot key aspects of the hand hygiene program if the compliance rate falls.

Setting Aims

Dramatic improvement requires setting clear aims and quantitative time-specific improvement targets. An organization will not improve without a firm commitment and measurable goals. Teams are more successful when they have unambiguous, focused aims. Setting numerical goals clarifies the aims, creates tension for change, directs measurement, and focuses initial changes. Once aims have been established, the team needs to be careful not to back away from the aims deliberately or "drift" away unconsciously. Appropriate resources and personnel time must be allocated to achieve raise-the-bar targets.

An example of an appropriate aim for improving hand hygiene compliance can be as modest as, "Increase hand hygiene compliance by 25% within one year." However, more aggressive targets are desirable. Consistent with the JCAHO's National Patient Safety Goal #7, a raise-the-bar aim would be to improve hand hygiene compliance to greater than 90%. This latter goal helps change the focus from hand hygiene as a laudable practice to hand hygiene as a mandatory procedure. Regardless of the exact numeric target, the aim should be endorsed completely and enthusiastically by institutional leadership and opinion leaders.

Using the Model for Improvement

In order to move this work forward in your organization, IHI recommends using the Model for Improvement. Developed by Associates in Process Improvement, the Model for Improvement is a simple yet powerful tool for accelerating improvement that has been used successfully by hundreds of health care organizations to improve many different health care processes and outcomes.

The model has two parts:

- Three fundamental questions that guide improvement teams to: 1) set clear aims; 2) establish measures that will tell if changes are leading to improvement; and 3) identify changes that are likely to lead to improvement.
- Plan-Do-Study-Act (PDSA) cycles—small-scale tests of change in real work settings. Teams plan a test, try it, observe the results, and act on what is learned. It is critical for tests to be small and rapid (e.g., a test with two intensive care unit patients tomorrow). This is the scientific method applied to action-oriented learning.

Implementation:

After testing a change on a small scale, learning from each test, and refining the change through several PDSA cycles, the team can implement the change on a broader scale—for example, try to determine the best location for alcohol-based hand hygiene products and gloves at the point of care in just one or two rooms in the ICU; try including checks on the availability of alcohol-based hand hygiene products and compliance with hand hygiene and glove policies in multidisciplinary rounds.

Spread:

After successful implementation of a change or package of changes for a pilot population or an entire unit, the team can spread the changes to other parts of the organization or to other organizations.

You can learn more about the Model for Improvement and how to spread improvements on IHI's website [http://www.IHI.org/IHI/Topics/Improvement].

Getting Started

Do not expect that the hand hygiene and glove intervention package can be implemented successfully overnight. A successful program involves careful planning, testing to determine if the processes are working, making modifications as needed, retesting, and carefully implementing best practices.

- Select the team and the ward(s) for initial testing of change ideas.
- Assess current practice and compliance. Even if there is a hand hygiene and glove program currently in place, work with staff to begin preparing for changes to achieve raise-the-bar performance targets. Perform a survey to determine baseline hand hygiene and glove compliance rates. Determine how these compliance rates compare to those published in the literature.
- Organize an educational program. Teach the core principles of hand hygiene and glove practices to clinical staff throughout the hospital. Providing feedback to staff using baseline compliance data will open people's minds to opportunities for improvement.
- Assess satisfaction with current hand hygiene products. If an alcohol-based hand hygiene product is already available in the institution, interview caregivers about their satisfaction with the product in terms of degree of skin irritation, consistency ("stickiness"), drying time, scent, and ease of use and reliability of dispensers.
- If an alcohol-based hand hygiene product is not currently available in the institution, have nurses and some physicians trial two or three products to determine which one(s) are most acceptable to clinical staff before selecting the product to be used. It is also important to evaluate the design and function of dispensers before selecting a product for use since poorly functioning dispensers may adversely affect hand hygiene compliance rates.
- Solicit input from clinical staff (including nurses, physicians, respiratory therapists, and others on the care team) about the best locations for installing alcohol-based hand hygiene product dispensers.
- Introduce the hand hygiene intervention package to all staff.

First Test of Change

Once a team has prepared the way for change by studying the current process and educating health care providers, the next step is to begin testing the hand hygiene intervention package.

- Select a few nursing units on which to begin using the intervention package.

- Make sure that alcohol-based hand hygiene product dispensers have been installed at the point of care and are functioning properly.
- Ensure that there is an adequate supply of clean gloves of various sizes available at the point of care.
- Conduct educational sessions on individual nursing units, or sessions that can be attended by personnel from multiple nursing units. Include patient care managers in early educational sessions.
- Give demonstrations on the appropriate techniques for using an alcohol-based hand rub and handwashing with soap and water.
- Have a member of the team (e.g., an infection control professional) visit the nursing unit(s) to answer any questions about using an alcohol-based hand hygiene product routinely for cleansing hands and appropriate use of gloves.
- Place hand hygiene promotion posters in highly visible locations throughout the hospital and begin a multi-modal campaign to improve performance.
- Engage patients and families by providing a patient safety "tip sheet," including information about hand hygiene best practices. Encourage patients and families to remind clinical staff to comply with hand hygiene and glove policies.

Measurement

Measurement tools have been included as appendices in this guide:
- Appendix 1. Hand Hygiene Knowledge Assessment Questionnaire
- Appendix 2. Checklist for the Availability of Alcohol-Based Hand Rub and Clean Gloves
- Appendix 3. Hand Hygiene and Glove Use Monitoring Form

For Appendices 2 and 3, please refer to the forms for specific information regarding the recommended process and outcome measures for improving hand hygiene.

Compliance with all aspects of each of the four interventions in the hand hygiene package should be measured as "all-or-none." In other words, if staff demonstrate correct knowledge of some, but not all, of the aspects of hand hygiene and glove use, they are not in compliance with the intervention package. If staff demonstrate only partial competency, they are not yet competent. If alcohol is present at the point of care but the dispenser is empty or gloves are not available, this is not compliant with the package. Similarly, all aspects of hand hygiene and glove use must be performed correctly during a patient encounter. This measurement strategy recognizes that raise-the-bar performance requires highly reliable care processes, and that from the patient's point of view, partial compliance is unacceptable.

Measurement is the only way to know whether a change represents an improvement. There are a number of measures that can be used to determine if hand hygiene and glove use are improving.

> ***1. The percentage of caregivers who answer all five questions correctly on a standardized hand hygiene knowledge assessment survey***
>
> This measure assesses the proportion of clinical staff who demonstrate adequate knowledge of the key elements of hand hygiene and glove use. A simple, rapid, and low technology strategy is to assess the knowledge of caregivers in real time on the ward. Consider selecting a random sample of 10 clinical providers from diverse disciplines each month (or at other intervals specified by the hospital) to answer a five-question survey (see Appendix 1) in tandem with a competency check (see measure 2 below). Specific questions can be designated by the hospital and/or selected from examples in the survey in Appendix 1.
>
> An alternative strategy is to assess knowledge using an Intranet-based learning or knowledge management system. Such electronic systems are being adopted rapidly by health care institutions in the United States. The clear advantage of this approach is that the entire clinical staff can be tested annually, or a sample may be tested at more frequent intervals. Completion of the assessment can be documented electronically and used for recredentialing purposes. Some systems can document which questions are being answered incorrectly, allowing direct measurement of the percent of caregivers who answer all of the questions correctly and facilitating design of targeted educational programs. However, some systems do not capture incorrect answers, and others allow personnel to retake the test as often as necessary to achieve a perfect score, making it impossible to calculate the required measure.
>
> ***2. The percentage of caregivers who perform all three key hand hygiene procedures correctly***
>
> This is a simple, rapid, low technology strategy that can be used in tandem with the method described in measure 1. Randomly select a sample of 10 clinical providers from diverse disciplines each month (or at other intervals specified by the hospital) and observe them to determine if they perform the three key hand hygiene procedures correctly: handwashing, alcohol-based hand rub, and gloves. This method has the strength of direct evaluation and feedback, but is time consuming. It also provides an opportunity to ensure that providers are not wearing artificial nails or nail extenders and have their nails trimmed to less than ¼ inch.
>
> > ➢ Boyce JM, Pittet D. Guideline for Hand Hygiene in Health-Care Settings: Recommendations of the Healthcare Infection Control Practices Advisory Committee and the HICPAC/SHEA/APIC/IDSA Hand Hygiene Task Force. *Morbid Mortal Wkly Rep.* 2002;51:1-45.
>
> Alternatively, competence can be assessed by monitoring hand hygiene practices during actual work (see measure 4 below). This has the advantage of being unobtrusive and integrated with other monitoring activities, but precludes direct feedback and adds complexity to the monitoring process.
> - Handwashing: Wash hands with soap and water, including contact with soap for at least 15 seconds, covering all surfaces (palm, back of hand, fingers, fingertips, and fingernails); rub with friction

- Turn off water without recontaminating hands: If the faucet is hand-operated, use paper towel to turn off the faucet; if the faucet is automatic, credit for compliance is given for correct performance
  - Dry hands with fresh paper towel
- Alcohol-based hand hygiene product (rub, gel, or foam): Use enough to cover all surfaces (palm, back of hand, fingers, fingertips, and fingernails); rub until dry (at least 15 seconds), which ensures sufficient volume has been applied
- Remove gloves using correct technique (so as not to contaminate the hands with a contaminated glove surface)

3. The percentage of bed spaces at which there are clean gloves in appropriate sizes and dispensers (wall-mounted or free-standing bottles) for alcohol-based hand rub/gel/foam that contain product, are functional, and dispense an appropriate volume of product

Make direct observations monthly (or at other intervals specified by the hospital) using a standardized procedure and form (see Appendix 2) on the same nursing units where measures 1 and 2 are monitored. Alternatively, availability can be assessed periodically as part of routine multidisciplinary rounds.

- Dispenser of alcohol-based product must be present, readily accessible at the point of care, not empty, functional, and capable of delivering the appropriate volume of product. If hand/pocket bottles are used, an adequate supply must be readily available and accessible on the ward.
- At least two sizes of gloves should be available and readily accessible at the point of care.

4. The percentage of patient encounters in which there is compliance by health care workers with all components of appropriate hand hygiene and glove practices

Compliance is monitored with direct observation by a trained observer using a standardized procedure and form (see Appendix 3). Independent observers are strongly recommended, preferably individuals who routinely are on the ward for other purposes and are not part of the care team. (This independent monitoring can be reinforced with monitoring by the care team during routine multidisciplinary rounds, which permits immediate assessment and feedback.) Observation periods should be 20-30 minutes (repeated if necessary) so that approximately 25-30 patient encounters are observed. The emphasis should be on observing complete encounters so that the proper measure of *complete* compliance with all components of the hand hygiene and glove intervention package can be calculated. Divide the number of encounters in which all components were performed correctly by the number of encounters observed and multiply by 100 to calculate the percentage compliance rate.

"Complete compliance" is defined by the adherence with the hand hygiene techniques and use of gloves as outlined in the table below. Gloves should be worn for all types of contact if the patient is on isolation precautions that require the use of gloves for contact with the patient and the environment, or if there is a unit-based procedure for universal gloving (wearing gloves for contact with all patients and their immediate environment).

Type of contact	Hand hygiene before	Hand hygiene after	Use of gloves
Patient contact that involves an invasive procedure (i.e., insertion of an intravascular catheter, urinary catheter, or other invasive device)	Yes	Yes	Yes
Patient contact that involves direct contact or potential contact with blood, body fluids, secretions (except sweat), excretions, mucous membranes, and nonintact skin (i.e., wounds, ulcers)	Yes	Yes	Yes
Patient contact not involving those noted above (i.e., taking vital signs, examination, repositioning, etc.)	Yes	Yes	*
Contact with the patient environment	—	Yes	*

Gloves should be worn for all types of contact if the patient is on isolation precautions that require the use of gloves for contact with the patient and the environment, or if there is a unit-based procedure for universal gloving (wearing gloves for contact with all patients and their immediate environment).

The following additional measure can also be used, but it does not replace direct observation of health care worker compliance during patient encounters:

- Volume of alcohol-based hand hygiene product consumed per week (or per month) divided by the number of patient days in the corresponding time period

Self-reporting by personnel or patients is not a reliable measure of compliance.

Barriers That May Be Encountered

- **Reluctance to change, tolerance of the status quo:** All change is difficult. The antidote is knowledge about the deficiencies of the present process and optimism about the potential benefits of a new process. The rate of compliance in most institutions is woeful, and dramatic improvement is possible.
- **Lack of leadership commitment and follow-through:** Hard work and good intentions cannot produce dramatic, long-term change without leadership buy-in and support.
- **Failure to educate and communicate:** Staff must understand the rationale for hand hygiene and glove practices, the danger of non-compliance to themselves and their patients, and the effectiveness and tolerability of hand hygiene products.
- **Failure to tailor product selection to staff preferences:** Staff should test products before they are introduced.

- **Lack of staff self-efficacy and empowerment:** Staff must believe that they have the ability and power to make major improvements.
- **Failure to make compliance a social norm and establish a culture of safety:** Staff must be empowered to remind other caregivers, regardless of rank or position, to practice hand hygiene. This should be reinforced by patients.
- **Failure to provide real time feedback of performance data:** Performance data should be communicated regularly and properly. Post trended data prominently.
- **Lack of a cohesive approach to behavior change:** A multi-factorial, creative approach to behavior change is essential.
- **Lack of physician buy-in:** Opinion leaders, role models, and physician champions, armed with educational materials and evidence, are essential.

APPENDIX ONE
Hand Hygiene
Knowledge Assessment
Questionnaire

Use this questionnaire to periodically survey clinical staff about their knowledge of key elements of hand hygiene. Select 5 questions from this survey, or use other questions derived from your hospital's existing educational program. *[NOTE: The correct answer for each question has been indicated below.]*

1. In which of the following situations should hand hygiene be performed? *[Correct answer: #4]*
   A. Before having direct contact with a patient
   B. Before inserting an invasive device (e.g., intravascular catheter, foley catheter)
   C. When moving from a contaminated body site to a clean body site during an episode of patient care
   D. After having direct contact with a patient or with items in the immediate vicinity of the patient
   E. After removing gloves

Circle the number for the best answer:
   1. B and E
   2. A, B and D
   3. B, D and E
   4. All of the above

2. If hands are not visibly soiled or visibly contaminated with blood or other proteinaceous material, which of the following regimens is the most effective for reducing the number of pathogenic bacteria on the hands of personnel? *[Correct answer: C]*

Circle the letter corresponding to the single best answer:
   A. Washing hands with plain soap and water
   B. Washing hands with an antimicrobial soap and water
   C. Applying 1.5 ml to 3 ml of alcohol-based hand rub to the hands and rubbing hands together until they feel dry

3. How are antibiotic-resistant pathogens most frequently spread from one patient to another in health care settings? *[Correct answer: C]*

Circle the letter corresponding to the single best answer:
   A. Airborne spread resulting from patients coughing or sneezing
   B. Patients coming in contact with contaminated equipment
   C. From one patient to another via the contaminated hands of clinical staff
   D. Poor environmental maintenance

4. Which of the following infections can be potentially transmitted from patients to clinical staff if appropriate glove use and hand hygiene are not performed? *[Correct answer: E]*

Circle the letter corresponding to the single best answer:
   A. Herpes simplex virus infection
   B. Colonization or infection with methicillin-resistant *Staphylococcus aureus*
   C. Respiratory syncytial virus infection
   D. Hepatitis B virus infection
   E. All of the above

5. *Clostridium difficile* (the cause of antibiotic-associated diarrhea) is readily killed by alcohol-based hand hygiene products. *[Correct answer: False]*

   ___ True
   ___ False

6. Which of the following pathogens readily survive in the environment of the patient for days to weeks? *[Correct answer: #3]*
   A. *E. coli*
   B. *Klebsiella spp.*
   C. *Clostridium difficile* (the cause of antibiotic-associated diarrhea)
   D. Methicillin-resistant *Staphyloccus aureus* (MRSA)
   E. Vancomycin-resistant enterococcus (VRE)

Circle the number for the best answer:
   1. A and D
   2. A and B
   3. C, D, E
   4. All of the above

7. Which of the following statements about alcohol-based hand hygiene products is accurate? *[Correct answer: C]*

Circle the letter corresponding to the single best answer:
   A. They dry the skin more than repeated handwashing with soap and water
   B. They cause more allergy and skin intolerance than chlorhexidine gluconate products
   C. They cause stinging of the hands in some providers due to pre-existing skin irritation
   D. They are effective even when the hands are visibly soiled
   E. They kill bacteria less rapidly than chlorhexidine gluconate and other antiseptic containing soaps

APPENDIX TWO

Checklist for the Availability of Alcohol-Based Hand Rub and Clean Gloves

Instructions:

1. Each row should be used to record data regarding the availability of an alcohol-based hand rub (liquid, gel, or foam) and clean gloves at the point of care for an individual patient. A point of care is a bedspace, exam room, or treatment/procedure area. If multiple hand rub bottles or dispensers are available at a specific point of care, only one need be assessed. If pocket/belt bottles or dispensers are the primary way hand rub is dispensed in the unit or department, each row should be used to assess the bottle or dispenser for an individual health care worker providing care to patients in this unit or department during the assessment period.

2. The room number and bedspace fields are used to facilitate a complete assessment of all points of care in a unit or department and for reference if problems are noted with the availability of hand-rub bottles or dispensers or clean gloves, or if additional comments are recorded.

3. To qualify as being near the patient, a hand-rub bottle or dispenser and clean gloves should be accessible to a health care worker who is standing or sitting at the point of care (i.e., close to the patient's bed or attached to the frame of the bed) or to a health care worker who approaches the point of care (i.e., inside the patient's room just inside the door or in the corridor adjacent to door).

4. For the purposes of this measurement exercise, each bottle or dispenser should be assessed with regard to its capacity to dispense the correct volume into the hand of the user when activated once (i.e., that the bottle is not empty, is functional and does not spray aberrantly, and dispenses correct volume of product). Additional comments regarding bottles that are poorly placed, nearly empty, or functioning incorrectly can be noted in the comments section of the form to facilitate remedial action.

5. Codes are: Y = Yes, N = No.

6. In the Adherence field, use the following rule: Y = if **all** elements are Y (that is, Near patient, Not empty, Functional, Dispenses correct volume, and Clean gloves near patient are **all** Y); N = if not.

7. Count the total number of Y for each column and record the total in box at the bottom of each column.

8. Calculate the percent adherence using the formula below and record the percent in the box at the bottom of each column. Total # of Y ÷ Total # of Points of Care (number of rows with data recorded) x 100

Checklist for the Availability of Alcohol-Based Hand Rub and Clean Gloves

Unit/Dept.: _________________________   Day of Week: _______   Date: ____/____/____   Time: ___:___AM/PM to ___:___AM/PM Initials _______

Room #	Bedspace #	Hand rub bottle or dispenser			Dispenses correct volume	Clean gloves near patient	Adherence to all elements	Comments
		Near patient	Not empty	Functional				
1		Y N	Y N	Y N	Y N	Y N	Y N	
2		Y N	Y N	Y N	Y N	Y N	Y N	
3		Y N	Y N	Y N	Y N	Y N	Y N	
4		Y N	Y N	Y N	Y N	Y N	Y N	
5		Y N	Y N	Y N	Y N	Y N	Y N	
6		Y N	Y N	Y N	Y N	Y N	Y N	
7		Y N	Y N	Y N	Y N	Y N	Y N	
8		Y N	Y N	Y N	Y N	Y N	Y N	
9		Y N	Y N	Y N	Y N	Y N	Y N	
10		Y N	Y N	Y N	Y N	Y N	Y N	
11		Y N	Y N	Y N	Y N	Y N	Y N	
12		Y N	Y N	Y N	Y N	Y N	Y N	
13		Y N	Y N	Y N	Y N	Y N	Y N	
14		Y N	Y N	Y N	Y N	Y N	Y N	
15		Y N	Y N	Y N	Y N	Y N	Y N	
16		Y N	Y N	Y N	Y N	Y N	Y N	
17		Y N	Y N	Y N	Y N	Y N	Y N	
18		Y N	Y N	Y N	Y N	Y N	Y N	
19		Y N	Y N	Y N	Y N	Y N	Y N	
20		Y N	Y N	Y N	Y N	Y N	Y N	
21		Y N	Y N	Y N	Y N	Y N	Y N	
22		Y N	Y N	Y N	Y N	Y N	Y N	
23		Y N	Y N	Y N	Y N	Y N	Y N	
24		Y N	Y N	Y N	Y N	Y N	Y N	
25		Y N	Y N	Y N	Y N	Y N	Y N	
26		Y N	Y N	Y N	Y N	Y N	Y N	
27		Y N	Y N	Y N	Y N	Y N	Y N	
28		Y N	Y N	Y N	Y N	Y N	Y N	
29		Y N	Y N	Y N	Y N	Y N	Y N	
30		Y N	Y N	Y N	Y N	Y N	Y N	
	Total # Y							
	% Present	%	%	%	%	%	%	

APPENDIX THREE

Hand Hygiene and Glove Use Monitoring Form

Instructions:

1. Each row should be used to record an encounter between one healthcare worker (HCW) and one patient that involves touching by the HCW of the patient or the patient's immediate environment. In situations involving and extended or complicated encounter, it is appropriate to use more than one row (see #4 below). Encounters that do not involve touching (i.e., only verbal communication between the HCW and the patient) should not be recorded.

2. An encounter may involve patient contact, environmental contact or both.

3. Patient contact involves touching the patient's body, gown, or clothes. Environmental contact involves touching the patient's bed or bed linen, bedside equipment, or other equipment, supplies, articles, or surfaces in the patient's bedspace or room.

4. For the purposes of this measurement exercise, an encounter begins when a healthcare worker enters the patient's room or approaches the patient's bedside (for multibed rooms) and ends when the healthcare worker leaves the room or bedside. In a situation where a patient requires extended or complicated care (such as in an ICU), an encounter may involve multiple contacts and it may be appropriate to record these individually if they are distinct activities. For example, a nurse may perform multiple patient care tasks at the bedside, complete this care, and then begin a series of contacts with the patient's environment. Or a nurse may complete a task that involves contact with mucous membranes and secretions, such as suctioning a patient, and then take on a separate task at a separate body site, such as changing a dressing. To the extent that these contacts can be observed and distinguished clearly, they may be recorded separately on separate rows.

5. The observer must be aware of whether a patient is on any type of isolation precautions that require the use of gloves. This information is necessary to determine whether gloves are required (see below).

6. For patient contact, the observer should be aware of the nature of the contact. This information is necessary to determine whether gloves are required (see below). It is important to distinguish three general subtypes of patient contact:

    a. contact that involves performing an invasive procedure (i.e., inserting an intravascular catheter or indwelling urinary catheter);

(instructions continue on page 194)

Hand Hygiene and Glove Use Monitoring Form

Unit/Dept.: ______________________ Day of Week: ______ Date: ____/____/____ Time: ___:___AM/PM to ___:___AM/PM Initials ______

#	Type of Healthcare Worker (circle only one)								Type of contact				Hand hygiene before			Gloves				Hand hygiene after			Adherence						
									Patient		Environment					Required		Used					Hand hygiene		Glove use			Overall	
1	D	N	TH	PH	XR	ES	TR	OT	Y	N	Y	N	Alc	HW	N	Y	N	Y	N	Alc	HW	N	Y	N	Y	N	NA	Y	N
2	D	N	TH	PH	XR	ES	TR	OT	Y	N	Y	N	Alc	HW	N	Y	N	Y	N	Alc	HW	N	Y	N	Y	N	NA	Y	N
3	D	N	TH	PH	XR	ES	TR	OT	Y	N	Y	N	Alc	HW	N	Y	N	Y	N	Alc	HW	N	Y	N	Y	N	NA	Y	N
4	D	N	TH	PH	XR	ES	TR	OT	Y	N	Y	N	Alc	HW	N	Y	N	Y	N	Alc	HW	N	Y	N	Y	N	NA	Y	N
5	D	N	TH	PH	XR	ES	TR	OT	Y	N	Y	N	Alc	HW	N	Y	N	Y	N	Alc	HW	N	Y	N	Y	N	NA	Y	N
6	D	N	TH	PH	XR	ES	TR	OT	Y	N	Y	N	Alc	HW	N	Y	N	Y	N	Alc	HW	N	Y	N	Y	N	NA	Y	N
7	D	N	TH	PH	XR	ES	TR	OT	Y	N	Y	N	Alc	HW	N	Y	N	Y	N	Alc	HW	N	Y	N	Y	N	NA	Y	N
8	D	N	TH	PH	XR	ES	TR	OT	Y	N	Y	N	Alc	HW	N	Y	N	Y	N	Alc	HW	N	Y	N	Y	N	NA	Y	N
9	D	N	TH	PH	XR	ES	TR	OT	Y	N	Y	N	Alc	HW	N	Y	N	Y	N	Alc	HW	N	Y	N	Y	N	NA	Y	N
10	D	N	TH	PH	XR	ES	TR	OT	Y	N	Y	N	Alc	HW	N	Y	N	Y	N	Alc	HW	N	Y	N	Y	N	NA	Y	N
11	D	N	TH	PH	XR	ES	TR	OT	Y	N	Y	N	Alc	HW	N	Y	N	Y	N	Alc	HW	N	Y	N	Y	N	NA	Y	N
12	D	N	TH	PH	XR	ES	TR	OT	Y	N	Y	N	Alc	HW	N	Y	N	Y	N	Alc	HW	N	Y	N	Y	N	NA	Y	N
13	D	N	TH	PH	XR	ES	TR	OT	Y	N	Y	N	Alc	HW	N	Y	N	Y	N	Alc	HW	N	Y	N	Y	N	NA	Y	N
14	D	N	TH	PH	XR	ES	TR	OT	Y	N	Y	N	Alc	HW	N	Y	N	Y	N	Alc	HW	N	Y	N	Y	N	NA	Y	N
15	D	N	TH	PH	XR	ES	TR	OT	Y	N	Y	N	Alc	HW	N	Y	N	Y	N	Alc	HW	N	Y	N	Y	N	NA	Y	N
16	D	N	TH	PH	XR	ES	TR	OT	Y	N	Y	N	Alc	HW	N	Y	N	Y	N	Alc	HW	N	Y	N	Y	N	NA	Y	N
17	D	N	TH	PH	XR	ES	TR	OT	Y	N	Y	N	Alc	HW	N	Y	N	Y	N	Alc	HW	N	Y	N	Y	N	NA	Y	N
18	D	N	TH	PH	XR	ES	TR	OT	Y	N	Y	N	Alc	HW	N	Y	N	Y	N	Alc	HW	N	Y	N	Y	N	NA	Y	N
19	D	N	TH	PH	XR	ES	TR	OT	Y	N	Y	N	Alc	HW	N	Y	N	Y	N	Alc	HW	N	Y	N	Y	N	NA	Y	N
20	D	N	TH	PH	XR	ES	TR	OT	Y	N	Y	N	Alc	HW	N	Y	N	Y	N	Alc	HW	N	Y	N	Y	N	NA	Y	N
21	D	N	TH	PH	XR	ES	TR	OT	Y	N	Y	N	Alc	HW	N	Y	N	Y	N	Alc	HW	N	Y	N	Y	N	NA	Y	N
22	D	N	TH	PH	XR	ES	TR	OT	Y	N	Y	N	Alc	HW	N	Y	N	Y	N	Alc	HW	N	Y	N	Y	N	NA	Y	N
23	D	N	TH	PH	XR	ES	TR	OT	Y	N	Y	N	Alc	HW	N	Y	N	Y	N	Alc	HW	N	Y	N	Y	N	NA	Y	N
24	D	N	TH	PH	XR	ES	TR	OT	Y	N	Y	N	Alc	HW	N	Y	N	Y	N	Alc	HW	N	Y	N	Y	N	NA	Y	N
25	D	N	TH	PH	XR	ES	TR	OT	Y	N	Y	N	Alc	HW	N	Y	N	Y	N	Alc	HW	N	Y	N	Y	N	NA	Y	N
26	D	N	TH	PH	XR	ES	TR	OT	Y	N	Y	N	Alc	HW	N	Y	N	Y	N	Alc	HW	N	Y	N	Y	N	NA	Y	N
27	D	N	TH	PH	XR	ES	TR	OT	Y	N	Y	N	Alc	HW	N	Y	N	Y	N	Alc	HW	N	Y	N	Y	N	NA	Y	N
28	D	N	TH	PH	XR	ES	TR	OT	Y	N	Y	N	Alc	HW	N	Y	N	Y	N	Alc	HW	N	Y	N	Y	N	NA	Y	N
29	D	N	TH	PH	XR	ES	TR	OT	Y	N	Y	N	Alc	HW	N	Y	N	Y	N	Alc	HW	N	Y	N	Y	N	NA	Y	N
30	D	N	TH	PH	XR	ES	TR	OT	Y	N	Y	N	Alc	HW	N	Y	N	Y	N	Alc	HW	N	Y	N	Y	N	NA	Y	N

	Total # of Y		
% Adherence	%	%	%

Type of Healthcare Worker: **D** = attending, fellow, resident, PA, med stud; **N** = nurse, aide, **TH** = therapist (RT, PT, OT); **PH** = phlebotomy/IV team; **XR** = radiology technician; **ES** = environmental services; **TR** = transporter; **OT** = other

Hand hygiene before/after: Alc = alcohol-based hand rub; HW = handwashing with soap and water; N = none

Gloves Required: Y if isolation requiring gloves or contact involves an invasive procedure or contact with blood, body fluids, secretions/excretions, mucous membranes, or non-intact skin; N if not

Adherence: **Hand hygiene** -- Y if patient contact and hand hygiene before and after are both Y or if environmental contact only and hand hygiene after is Y; N = if not / **Glove use** -- Y if Gloves Required and Used are both Y; N if Gloves Required is Y and Used is N; NA if Gloves Required is N / **Overall adherence** -- Y if Hand hygiene is Y and glove use is Y or NA; N if not

Hand Hygiene and Glove Use Monitoring Form

Instructions, continued

    b. contact that involves actual or potential contact with blood, body fluids, secretions (except sweat), excretions, mucous membranes or non-intact skin (i.e., suctioning an intubated patient, emptying a urinal or bedpan, changing an dressing on an open wound);

    c. other patient contact that does not qualify for a or b (i.e., measuring vital signs, examining a patient, repositioning a patient, etc.).

7. Use the following codes to record data (Note: Y = Yes, N = No, unless otherwise noted): Type of Healthcare Worker: D = attending physician, fellow, resident, physician's assistant, medical student; N = nurse, aide, TH = therapist (respiratory therapist, physical therapist, occupational therapist); PH = phlebotomy/IV team; XR = radiology technician; ES = environmental services; TR = transporter; OT = other; Hand hygiene before/after: Alc = alcohol-based hand rub (liquid, gel, or foam); HW = handwashing with soap and water; N = none; Gloves Required: Y if the patient is on any type of isolation precautions requiring gloves or the Type of Contact involved an invasive procedure or actual/potential contact with blood, body fluids, secretions/excretions, mucous membranes, or non-intact skin; N if not.

8. In the Adherence section, use the following rules to record Y or N for Hand Hygiene, Glove Use, and Overall Adherence: Hand hygiene: Y if the Type of Contact was patient contact and Hand hygiene before and after are both Y or if the Type of Contact was Environmental Contact only and Hand hygiene after is Y; N = if not; Glove use: Y if Gloves Required and Used are both Y; N if Gloves Required is Y and Used is N; NA if Gloves Required is N; Overall: Y if Hand hygiene is Y and Glove Use is Y or NA; N if not.

9. In the Adherence section, count the number of Y for Hand hygiene, Glove use, and Overall and record the total in box at the bottom of each column.

10. In the Adherence section, calculate the percent adherence using the formulas below and record the percent in the box at the bottom of each column Hand hygiene: Total # of Y ÷ Total # of Encounters (number of rows with data recorded) x 100 Glove use: Total # of Y ÷ [Total # of Encounters (number of rows with data recorded) – Total # of NA] x 100 Overall: Total # of Y ÷ Total # of Encounters (number of rows with data recorded) x 100

Infection Control Web Resources

from the International Federation of Infection Control

The following Web resources were gathered for use in *Information Resources in Infection Control*, Fourth Edition (Editor: Nizam Damani M.D., MBBS, MSc, FRCPI, FRCPath), due in 2006 from the International Federation of Infection Control (IFIC). The full document will be available online at IFIC's Web site: http://www.theific.org/publications.asp.

Evidence-Based Practice Sites

Name	*Web site*
Agency for Health Care Research and Quality	http://www.ahcpr.gov/clinic/epcix.htm
Evidence-Based Medicine Tool Kit	http://www.med.ualberta.ca/ebm/ebm.htm
Evidence-Based Practice Centers	http://www.ahrq.gov/clinic/epc/
Evidence-Based Practice in Infection Control	http://www.epic.tvu.ac.uk
National Guideline Clearing House	http://www.ngc.gov
National Institute for Clinical Evidence	http://www.nice.org.uk
Netting the Evidence	http://www.shef.ac.uk/~scharr/ir/netting/
National Resource for Infection Control	http://www.nric.org.uk/
Scottish Intercollegiate Guidelines Network (SIGN)	http://www.sign.ac.uk/
The Cochrane Collaboration	http://www.cochrane.org/
The Joanna Briggs Institute	http://www.joannabriggs.edu.au/about/home.php

Journals

Name	*Web site*
American Journal of Infection Control	http://www.mosby.com/ajic
Australian Journal of Infection Control	http://www.aica.org.au/docs/journal/index.asp
British Journal of Infection Control	http://www.icna.co.uk/public/bjic/index.htm
Canada Communicable Disease Report	http://www.phac-aspc.gc.ca/publicat/ccdr-rmtc/index.html
Canadian Journal of Infection Control	http://www.chica.org/inside_cjic_journal.html
Communicable Disease Report Weekly	http://www.hpa.org.uk/cdr/
Communicable Diseases and Public Health	http://www.hpa.org.uk/cdph/
Emerging Infectious Diseases	http://www.cdc.gov/ncidod/eid/index.htm
Eurosurveillance	http://www.eurosurveillance.org/index-02.asp
Hospital Infection Control	http://www.thomson.com/common/view_brand_overview.jsp?section=healthcare&body_include=/healthcare/brand_overviews/AHC_HospitalInfectionControl&page_mode=full&subsection=&secondary=nursing_pat_ed&subnav=healthcare_professionals&tertiary=&product_name=%0A%0AHospital_Infection_Control%0A%0A
Infection Control and Hospital Epidemiology	http://www.journals.uchicago.edu/ICHE/home.html
Infection Control Resource	http://www.infectioncontrolresourse.org
International Journal of Infection Control	http://www.theific.org
Journal of Hospital Infection	http://intl.elsevierhealth.com/journals/jhin/default.cfm
Morbidity & Mortality Weekly Report (MMWR)	http://www.cdc.gov/mmwr/
WHO Weekly Epidemiology Record	http://www.who.int/wer/en/

Organizations, Institutions, and Regulatory Bodies

Name	*Web site*
American College of Occupational and Environmental Medicine	http://www.acoem.org/
American Dental Association	http://www.ada.org
American Society for Microbiology	http://www.asm.org/
Association for the Advancement of Medical Instrumentation	http://www.aami.org/index.htm
Association of Medical Microbiologists, UK	http://www.amm.co.uk
Association of Medical Microbiology and Infectious Disease Canada	http://www.ammi.ca/the_society/index.php
Association of Perioperative Registered Nurses (AORN), USA	http://www.aorn.org
Association for Professionals in Infection Control and Epidemiology (APIC), USA	http://www.apic.org
Australian Infection Control Association	http://www.aica.org.au/
Baltic Network Infection Control (BALTICCARE)	http://www.balticcare.org/Links.htm
British Dental Association	http://www.bda-dentistry.org.uk/
British Travel Health Association	http://www.btha.org
Canadian Association for Clinical Microbiology and Infectious Diseases	http://www.cacmid.ca/
Centers for Disease Control and Prevention (CDC), USA	http://www.cdc.gov
Centre Nacional de Epidemiologia, Spain (CNE)	http://cne.isciii.es/
Communicable Disease Surveillance Centre, Northern Ireland	http://www.cdscni.org.uk/
Communicable Disease Surveillance & Response (WHO)	http://www.who.int/wer/en/
Community and Hospital Infection Control Association (CHICA), Canada	http://www.chica.org

Department of Health, England, UK	http://www.dh.gov.uk/Home/fs/en
Dutch Working party on Infection Prevention (WIP)	http://www.wip.nl
European Centre for Disease Prevention and Control (ECDC)	http://ec.europa.eu/health/ph_overview/strategy/ecdc/ecdc_en.htm
European Forum for Hospital Sterile Supply (EFHSS)	http://www.efhss.com/
European Operating Room Nurses Association (EORNA)	http://www.eorna.org
European Society of Clinical Microbiology and Infectious Diseases	http://www.escmid.org
Euro-Mediterranean Public Health Information System (EMPHIS)	http://www.emphis.org/
European Society for Paediatric Infectious Diseases	http://www.espid.org/
Food and Drug Administration (FDA), USA	http://www.fda.gov
Global Infectious Diseases and Epidemiology Network (GIDEON)	http://www.gideononline.com/
Hand Hygiene Resource Centre	http://www.handhygiene.org
Health Canada Disease Prevention and Control Guidelines	http://www.hc-sc.gc.ca/
Health Protection Agency (HPA), UK	http://www.hpa.org.uk/infections/default.htm
Hospital in Europe Link for Infection Infection Control through Surveillance (HELICS)	http://helics.univ-lyon1.fr/
Hospital Infection Society, UK	http://www.his.org.uk/
Infection Control Nurses Association (ICNA), UK	http://www.icna.co.uk/
Infectious Diseases Society of America	http://www.idsociety.org/
Infectious Diseases Societies Worldwide	http://www.idlinks.com/
Institute of Decontamination Sciences	http://www.idsc-uk.org/
International Federation of Infection Control (IFIC)	http://www.theific.org

International Health Care Worker Safety Center, USA	http://www.healthsystem.virginia.edu/internet/epinet/
International Scientific Forum for Home Hygiene (IFH)	http://www.ifh-homehygiene.org/2003/index.html
International Society for Infectious Diseases	http://www.isid.org
International Society of Travel Medicine	http://www.istm.org
Johns Hopkins University ABX Guide (Infectious diseases)	http://hopkins-abxguide.org/
Medical Devices Agency (MDA), UK	http://www.medical-devices.gov.uk
Medicine and Healthcare Products Regulatory Agency (MHRA)	http://www.mhra.gov.uk
Medline	http://medline.cos.com/
National Disease Surveillance Centre, Republic of Ireland	http://www.ndsc.ie
National Foundation for Infectious Diseases, USA	http://www.nfid.org/
National Institute for Health and Clinical Excellence, UK	http://www.nice.org.uk
National Institute for Public Health Surveillance, France	http://www.invs.sante.fr/
National Institutes of Health (NIH), US	http://www.nih.gov/
National Nosocomial Surveillance System (of the CDC), USA	http://www.cdc.gov/ncidod/dhqp/nnis_pubs.html
National Electronic Library of Infection, UK	http://www.neli.org.uk/
NHS Estates (Department of Health, UK)	http://www.dh.gov.uk/PolicyAndGuidance/OrganisationPolicy/EstatesAndFacilitiesManagement/fs/en
Occupational Safety & Health Administration (OSHA), USA	http://www.osha.gov
Public Health Agency of Canada	http://www.phac-aspc.gc.ca/new_e.html
Public Health Laboratory Services (PHLS), UK (Now Health Protection Agency)	http://www.hpa.org.uk/infections/topics
Robert Koch Institute, Germany	http://www.rki.de/

Royal College of Nursing, UK	http://www.rcn.org.uk/resources/mrsa/ healthcarestaff/resources.php
Health Protection Scotland (formerly Scottish Centre for Infection and Environmental Health)	http://www.hps.scot.nhs.uk/
Société Française d'Hygiène Hospitalière, France (SFHH)	http://sfhh.univ-lyon1.fr/
Society for Healthcare Epidemiology of America (SHEA), USA	http://www.shea-online.org
Statens Serum Institut, Denmark (SSI)	http://www.ssi.dk/sw379.asp
Surveillance of Nosocomial Infections in the Netherlands	http://www.prezies.nl/
Webber Training	http://webbertraining.com
World Health Organization (WHO)	http://www.who.int/

Index

J

Joint Commission International
  accreditation survey process, 49, 53–67
  international conferences on infection
    prevention and control, 17
  International Patient Safety Goals, 17,
    27–28, 41, 49, 67
  Patient Safety Practices resource
    center, 18
  Prevention and Control of Infections
    standards, 27–40
    compliance checklist on, 27, 28,
      161–168
    summary list on, 28–29
  response to infection prevention and
    control crisis, 16–18
Joint Commission International Center for
  Patient Safety, 17–18

K

Kitchen sanitation and food handling, 33,
  64, 128–129, 163
Knowledge, scientific, as basis of IPC
  program, 36
  compliance checklist on, 165
  IPC plan background information
    on, 93

L

Laboratory procedures, 30, 38
  individual tracers in, 59
  quality management and improvement
    system in, 27, 30
  in SARS surveillance, 153
  system tracers in, 63, 64, 65
  waste and hazardous material
    management in, 38
Laundry and linen management, 33,
  123, 125
  compliance checklist on, 163
  in emergency, 132
  system tracers in, 64
Laws and regulations as basis of IPC
  program, 36
  compliance checklist on, 165
  IPC plan background information on, 93
Leadership in IPC program, 35, 70–74
  determining priority risk factors, 89
  expectations on hand hygiene
    compliance, 117–118, 180
  financial benefits for, 70, 72
  IPC staff as, 73–74
  methods increasing support, 70, 71
  physicians as, 70, 73

  systems tracer in assessment of, 64–65
Link Nurse Program, 76
Literature review on infection risks and
  rates, 101

M

Maintaining effective IPC program, 111–135
Malaria, 99
Management of IPC program, 35–36, 75–76
  communication of monitoring results
    to, 37, 167
  compliance checklist on, 164–166
  continuous and proactive
    communication in, 35, 75–76
  coordination responsibilities in,
    35, 75, 165
  IPC staff responsibilities for, 74
  oversight role in, 35–36, 74–75, 76, 164
  qualifications of personnel in,
    35, 75, 164
  responsibilities in, 35, 75–76
  summary list of standards on, 28–29
  systems tracers in assessment of, 64–65
Mask use, 34
  compliance checklist on, 164
  in SARS outbreak, 151
Medical transport, infection prevention
    and control in, 27, 30, 38, 39
  system tracers in assessment of, 63
Medication management
  appropriate antibiotic use in, 118–122
  tracer on, 66
Meningitis, 6, 103
  staff exposure to, 122
Meningococcal infections, 5, 6–7, 58
  reporting requirements in, 103
Methicillin-resistant *Staphylococcus aureus*
    (MRSA) infections, 1, 17
  hand hygiene affecting incidence of, 174
  risk assessment in, 90
  surveillance for, 99
Mission statement of IPC program, 89, 93
Monitoring of infection risks and rates,
    36–37, 166–167. *See also* Data
    collection and surveillance on
    infection risks and rates
Mortuary area, 33, 163
Multidisciplinary team
  in evaluation of IPC program, 104
  in hand hygiene improvement
    program, 180
  in oversight of IPC program, 35–36,
    74–75
  in performance improvement, 81–82,
    112, 114

Purchase
JCI Publications
Globally

Joint Commission International publications are available through a number of sources, some of which might be closer to you than you think. You can order directly through any of our international representatives:

Brazil
Distributor: Ernesto Reichmann
Distribuidora de Livros (ERDL)
Rua Coronel Marques 335
03440-000 São Paulo–SP Brazil
Phone: +55 (11) 8124-1011
Fax: +55 (11) 6198-2122
rgm@erdl.com

Eastern Europe
Representative: Laszlo Horvath
Tinodi u. 31.
1047 Budapest, Hungary
Phone: +36-1-3703614
Fax: +36-1-3795842
laszloaw@axelero.hu

Korea
Representative: Sunhee Shin
Panmun Book Co; Ltd
Mok 1-dong, Yangchon-ku
Seoul, South Korea, 158-051
Phone: +82 2 2653 5131
Fax: +82 2 2653 2454
shshin@panmun.co.kr

Middle East
Representative: Bill Kennedy
Avicenna Partnership
P.O. Box 484
Oxford, OX2 9WQ, UK
Phone: +44-1-387-251 447
Fax: +44-1-387-247375
bill.kennedy@btinternet.com

Philippines
Representative: Tony P. Sagun
CRW Books
4 Topaz Road, Greenheights
Taytay, Rizal, Philippines
Phone: +63-632-660-5480
+63-632-660-8430
Fax: +63-632-660-0342
apsagun@amdg.com.ph

Singapore, Malaysia, and Indonesia
Distributor: APAC
70 Bendemeer Road #05-03
Hiap Huat House
Singapore 334490
Phone: +65-68447333
steven@apacmedia.com.sg

Switzerland, Austria, and Germany
Distributor: Swiss Association for
    Standardization
Burlistrasse 29
CH-8400 Winterhur Switzerland
Phone: +41 52 2245442
Fax: +41-52 2245438
judith.brandsberg@snv.ch

Taiwan
Representative: Shirley Chu
HO-CHI Book Publishing
322-2 Ankang Road
Neihu Dist; Taipei 114
Taiwan R.O.C.
Phone: +886-2-27940168
Fax: +886-2-27924702
hochi@ms12.hinet.net

United Arab Emirates
Distributor: Sharjah University Bookshop
P.O. Box 30965
King Faisal Street
Sharjah
United Arab Emirates
Tel.: 00971 6 5726001
Fax: 00971 6 5726003
Email: univbksh@emirates.net.ae

You can place orders directly by mail:
    Joint Commission International Publications
    P.O. Box 75751
    Chicago, IL 60675-5751
    U.S.A.

Or you can fax your orders to:
    +1-317-610-4022

Booksellers should specify desired method of shipment from the United States, e.g., surface freight or air freight. All surface freight charges within the United States (to the bookseller's designated freight forwarder) will be charged to the customer at actual cost.

For further information on products, ordering, and delivery, the Joint Commission Resources 2006 International Catalogue is available online in PDF format at http://www.jcrinc.com/jcrinternationalcatalogue

Your opinion counts!

We hope you have found this publication to be a useful and practical resource as you make improvements to your medication management processes.

Please take a few moments to provide us with your thoughts and suggestions regarding this book by logging on to:

http://www.surveymonkey.com/s.asp?u=84542651651

Thank you!